Ethnic Minority Elderly

A Task Force Report
of the
American Psychiatric Association

The American Psychiatric Association Task Force on Ethnic Minority Elderly

Kenneth M. Sakauye, M.D., *Chairman*
F. M. Baker, M.D., M.P.H.
Ranjit C. Chacko, M.D.
Richard G. Jimenez, M.D.
Herbert W. Nickens, M.D.
James W. Thompson, M.D.

John M. de Figueiredo, M.D., *Corresponding Member*
Spero Manson, *Consultant*

Ethnic Minority Elderly

A Task Force Report
of the
American Psychiatric Association

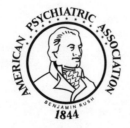

Published by the American Psychiatric Association
Washington, DC

Note: The authors have worked to ensure that all information in this book concerning drug dosages, schedules, and routes of administration is accurate as of the time of publication and consistent with standards set by the U.S. Food and Drug Administration and the general medical community. As medical research and practice advance, however, therapeutic standards may change. For this reason and because human and mechanical errors sometimes occur, we recommend that readers follow the advice of a physician who is directly involved in their care or the care of a member of their family.

The findings, opinions, and conclusions of this report do not necessarily represent the views of the officers, trustees, all members of the task force, or all members of the American Psychiatric Association. The views expressed are those of the authors of the individual chapters. Task force reports are considered a substantive contribution of the ongoing analysis and evaluation of problems, programs, issues, and practices in a given area of concern.

Copyright © 1994 American Psychiatric Association
ALL RIGHTS RESERVED
Manufactured in the United States of America on acid-free paper
First Edition
97 96 95 94   4 3 2 1

American Psychiatric Association
1400 K Street, N.W., Washington, DC   20005

Library of Congress Cataloging-in-Publication Data
American Psychiatric Association.   Task Force on Ethnic Minority
  Elderly.
    Ethnic minority elderly: a task force report of the American
  Psychiatric Association / [the American Psychiatric Association Task
  Force on Ethnic Minority Elderly].
      p.   cm.
    Includes bibliographical references and index.
    ISBN 0-89042-247-8 (alk. paper)
      1. Minority aged—Mental health services—United States—
  Evaluation. 2. Minority aged—Mental health services—United
  States—Planning. 3. Minority aged—Mental health services—United
  States—Abstracts. 4. Minority aged—Mental health—United States—
  Abstracts. I. Title.
    [DNLM: 1. Mental Health Service—in old age—United States.
  2. Minority Groups—United States. 3. Ethnic Groups—United States.
  4. Health Services Accessibility—United States. 5. Health Services
  Needs and Demand—United States.   WA 305 A512e 1994]
  RC451.5.A2A46 1994
  362.2'08'693—dc20
  DNLM/DLC
  for Library of Congress   93-27940
                                                                      CIP

British Library Cataloguing in Publication Data
A CIP record is available from the British Library.

Contents

Chapter 1

Executive Summary and Recommendations

Introduction

The American Psychiatric Association (APA) has long been concerned about the availability and adequacy of psychiatric services for minority populations. The APA Council on National Affairs' minority committees have both raised practitioner consciousness and broadened our understanding of many of the issues affecting minority patient and practitioner populations. However, in 1987, the APA Council on Aging became increasingly concerned that the minority elderly—a growing percentage of elders, including the "old-old," who survive to age 85 and beyond—have not received adequate attention in either clinical studies or practice, notwithstanding the common-sense dicta that the minority elderly face multiple jeopardies, have fewer resources, and, in many cases, are not within the cultural mainstream of service needs and delivery. This concern gave rise to the establishment of the Task Force on Ethnic Minority Elderly, approved by the APA Board of Trustees in 1988.

The task force was given a specific charge to gain further knowledge of the following: the needs of the mentally ill minority elderly, how to use existing (and develop new) service models to meet those needs, whether and how to incorporate issues about ethnic minority elderly populations into training curricula, and how to enhance psychiatrists' capacity to work with individuals in these populations.

The task force would do the following:

1. Define the scope of the problem (determine which populations constitute the ethnic minority elderly and set parameters for initial activities)

1

2. Explore existing epidemiologic and clinical literature on the ethnic minority elderly and prepare an annotated bibliography of this material
3. Establish a research agenda for addressing the psychiatric problems and adjustment difficulties of the ethnic minority elderly
4. Explore issues of service delivery (including the existence or development of segregated services) and propose mechanisms to enhance the suitability of all existing services
5. Define issues that ethnic minority groups see as central to efforts to sensitize psychiatrists to the needs of these populations
6. Make recommendations for training in ethnic minority issues within general and specialized geriatric psychiatry curricula
7. Identify existing psychiatrists who are involved in treatment of minority elderly patients and systematically examine their experiences (most clinicians working with these populations are not working in academic settings and do not generally publish their findings); this would form the basis for the development of a directory of such individuals for use by district branches and minority organizations
8. Work with the APA components involved with international medical graduates and minorities to help enhance the training of bilingual, culturally aware psychiatrists to work with the minority elderly
9. Work with the Joint Commission on Public Affairs to develop mechanisms of outreach to the minority elderly populations in need of service, bearing in mind cultural issues such as translation and reverse bias against psychiatry

This report represents the product of the task force's deliberation and research into mental health issues confronting the ethnic minority elderly, and underscores the wide gaps in knowledge and understanding of these diverse populations and their mental health statuses and needs. We make a series of recommendations for action at the federal, state, and psychiatric-community levels to begin to address the psychiatric needs of the ethnic minority elderly.

The Nature of the Problem

Although two White House Conferences on Aging and other national entities have made specific recommendations addressing minority mental health issues, little action has actually been visible. In part, the inattention to ethnic diversity among the elderly reflects the misconception that the problem of the ethnic minority elderly reflects simply their "culture of poverty." In the main, noneconomic cultural elements have received less public attention. Moreover, the degree of "ethnic influence" varies widely, increasing with each new generation and its greater assimilation to and acceptance in mainstream society. Today, increased sensitivity to the importance of cultural differences and needs has been met by a backlash against many ethnic and racial groups. Increased racial incidents, overt racial polarization, and sentiments against continuing many entitlement programs have reappeared. Even in education, the media provide increasing numbers of reports of professionals who denounce both teaching or reviewing their areas of educational expertise from a minority point of view, claiming that to do so is a repressive attempt to force politically correct interpretations.

For many years, minority groups themselves have resisted being the subjects of study. The experience of prejudice and mistreatment, real or perceived, remains strong. The fear and suspicion about being a subject of study remain high. Many individuals in minority groups fear that probing into their ethnic origins may unleash unhealthy racist prejudices and foster renewed discrimination. Such concerns, at one time, led to efforts to abolish questions about race in governmental statistical surveys.

Despite these barriers and impediments to study, we must strive to evaluate possible racial differences both in rates of incidence of mental illness and in responses to biological treatments and psychotherapeutic approaches. To improve diagnosis and care, we must consider the social setting and cultural group expectations that account for gaps in research, low service use by minority elders, differing levels of knowledge about mental illness, and differing etiologies of particular health and mental health problems. For example, if the prevalence of mental illness, in fact, is lower in certain minority elderly groups because of the "survivor effect"— only the most physically and mentally healthy living to old age—then the need for early health promotion and intervention strategies is highlighted. Low service use by the minority elderly may be ascribed more to financial barriers, inadequate knowledge of service opportunities, or perceived or real absence of high-quality care than to an absence of identifiable mental illness or a group preference for alternative care mechanisms.

To begin to meet its charge, the task force surveyed research on health services for, and clinical literature on the mental health of, ethnic minority elderly populations. The task force sought to determine the various positions and opinions about the mental health needs of these populations, as well as the level of support for them by the clinical care community and policy making groups. References gleaned from this literature survey are presented in the chapter sections on specific minority-population issues, in annotated bibliographic form, as well as at the end of the volume in Appendix 1. Because the task force's focus is on psychiatric problems, only the most relevant commentaries, editorials, or other material from the larger body of anthropological and sociological data on ethnic minority elderly are included. As presented in Chapter 2, Dr. James Thompson of the University of Maryland Department of Psychiatry reanalyzed the National Institute of Mental Health (NIMH)–funded Epidemiologic Catchment Area (ECA) data for rates of mental illness, thus providing the most extensive information available on gross rates of mental illness in minority elderly populations.

General Findings

The growth of minority populations, and elderly minority in particular, is leading to a demographic imperative to deal with the questions raised (see Tables 1–1 through 1–3). Relevant studies were limited in both number and scope; indeed, for some ethnic groups, no research has appeared in the literature. In many instances, the task force was forced to extrapolate from studies of younger adults, which is an imperfect method at best. Impressions gleaned by the task force from ethnic community mental health workers and leaders largely support the commentaries in the individual chapters.

General Research Themes

Available data confirm that the mental health problems and needs of minority elderly are, for the most part, neither well recognized nor well served. A number of general themes emerged for consideration in both the public policy sector and psychiatric community:

Table 1–1. 1990 U.S. population for all ages and for elderly, by minority group

Population (in thousands)	All ages			Elderly				
	Total	Male	Female	65–74	75–84	≥85	Percentage of minority group	Percentage of U.S. elderly
U.S. total	248,710	121,239	127,470	18,106	10,055	3,080	—	12.6
White	199,686	97,476	102,210	15,226	9,038	2,788	13.55	86.6
African American	29,986	14,170	15,816	1,503	774.9	230.2	8.37	8.0
Hispanic[a]	22,354	11,388	10,966	723.0	343.7	94.6	5.2	3.7
Asian/Pacific Islander	7,274	3,558	3,716	300.7	124.0	29.7	6.2	1.4
Native American	1,959	967	992	72.0	33.3	9.2	5.8	0.8

Note. The total of all ethnic groups exceeds the U.S. total population because some Hispanic figures overlap white, African American, and Native American counts.
[a]Refer to Table 4–1 for Hispanic census data.
Source. United States Bureau of the Census: *1990 Census of Population and Housing Summary, Tape File 1C.* Washington, DC, U.S. Department of Commerce, 1991.

1. With the exception of African Americans, American Indians, and Alaska and Hawaiian natives, many minority elders are new immigrants, arriving in the United States in old age, to be reunited with their children who have paved the way. This group experiences the greatest culture shock and has the least chance of assimilation. Such individuals frequently are isolated, maintaining different cultural values and habits. They present culture-bound syndromes and diagnostic difficulties, and then face language and financial barriers to treatment. Although underlying issues are similar for all new immigrants, each ethnic group poses unique sets of problems. Test validity, language, family networks, and available resources differ for each group.

2. Less-recent immigrants seem to have fewer mental health problems than the newly arrived. When the fact or recency of immigration is not the issue, prejudice toward or segregation of the ethnic minority affects family life, social networks, self-esteem, access to and choices in care, and attitudes—in ways that are separate and distinct from problems caused by the "culture of poverty." Workers who deal with these populations must be taught sensitivity to the unique issues and characteristics of, and issues confronting, various ethnic groups, whether recent immigrants or long-time residents.

3. Segregated care has again become a fact of life for ethnic minority elderly populations, although today it stems from intentions wholly different from those of the past. Concerned public policy makers have

Table 1–2. U.S. Hispanic population in 1990, by place of origin

Hispanics	Total U.S. Population	Percentage of Hispanics
Mexican	13,421,000	62.6
Puerto Rican	2,382,000	11.1
Cuban	1,055,000	4.9
Central or South American	2,951,000	13.8
Other Hispanic	1,628,000	7.6
Total	21,437,000	100.00
Non-Hispanics	226,355,814	—

Note. Table includes African American, white, and mixed Native American overlap.

Table 1–3. Elderly U.S. population in 1990, by race group

Group	Men	Women	Total	Percentage of elders
Hispanic				
65–74	315,383	407,646	723,029	62.26
75–84	132,529	211,161	343,690	29.60
≥ 85	33,497	61,067	94,564	8.14
All elders	481,409	679,874	1,161,283	100
Percentage elderly	41.45%	58.55%	5.20% of Hispanics 3.72% of all U.S. elderly	
African American				
65–74	617,641	885,819	1,503,460	59.93
75–84	279,199	495,709	774,908	30.89
≥ 85	68,592	161,591	230,183	9.18
All elders	965,432	1,543,119	2,508,551	100
Percentage elderly	38.49%	61.51%	8.37% of African Americans 8.03% of all U.S. elderly	
Asian				
65–74	133,818	166,913	300,731	66.17
75–84	58,230	65,759	123,989	27.28
≥ 85	12,399	17,339	29,738	6.54
All elders	204,447	250,011	454,458	100
Percentage elderly	44.99%	55.01%	6.25% of Asians 1.45% of all U.S. elderly	
Native American				
65–74	31,798	40,182	71,980	62.89
75–84	13,017	20,251	33,268	29.07
≥ 85	3,274	5,931	9,205	8.04
All elders	48,089	66,364	114,453	100
Percentage elderly	42.02%	57.98%	5.84% of Native Americans 0.37% of all U.S. elderly	
White				
65–74	7,068,958	8,157,243	15,226,201	56.28
75–84	3,381,501	5,656,219	9,037,720	33.41
≥ 85	764,450	2,023,602	2,788,052	10.31
All white elders	11,214,909	15,837,064	27,051,973	100
Percentage elderly	41.46	58.54	13.55% of whites 86.59% of all U.S. elderly	

suggested that culture-fair programs—whether for mental health or long-term care—require special ethnic services that cannot be supplied through mainstream programs. Such well-meaning reverse discrimination raises significant public policy questions warranting special study.

Population-Specific Themes

African American elderly. The African American elderly may well be overdiagnosed with schizophrenia and dementia, in part because of nontraditional presenting complaints and potential stereotyping by health care professionals. Dietary and life-style differences and a higher rate of alcoholism have increased the health risks of the African American elderly for cerebrovascular disease and chronic physical illnesses that strain the support network and increase mental health problems.

The historical context of exclusion of African Americans from the health care and educational systems has caused the African American elderly to have less knowledge of and trust in the formal care system, effectively continuing their exclusion. Even many middle-class African American families and the sizable new immigrant population still underuse the traditional health and mental health care community. Fortunately, the strong extended kinship network that extends beyond the nuclear family is a unique feature of the African American community that serves as strong support for the elderly member.

Asian American elderly. The prototypical close-knit and successful Asian family, complete with revered elder, belies significant intergenerational strain and socioeconomic differences. Older immigrants whose families came before the Asian Exclusion Act of 1917 are largely American born and highly economically assimilated. Rates of mental illness and suicide are largely unknown for this group, but appear higher than previously thought. The new immigrating elderly individual, joining children who paved the way, may experience significant adjustment problems. Many refugee families have had particularly difficult adjustments because they were poorly educated, were highly superstitious, came to cities from rural backgrounds, and had minimal resources when they arrived. Unfortunately, due to language and financial barriers, cultural differences, fear of inappropriate psychotropic medication use and misdiagnosis, such individuals do not make use of formal care systems, thereby excluding themselves from high quality medical intervention.

Hispanic American elderly.   The diversity of Hispanic populations in the United States, their continuous immigration over two centuries, and the high rate of intermarriage with other groups have made it difficult to iterate specific characteristics of all members of this ethnic minority population. In general, however, problems have arisen in the assessment and treatment of bilingual or non-English speaking individuals. With this group, the validity of existing screening instruments has been questioned; language barriers and cultural attitudes have led to misdiagnosis and underuse of traditional services. Hispanic Americans face higher rates of diabetes, obesity, alcoholism, and, possibly, earlier disability. True rates of depression or other forms of mental illness have not been well established, although they may rise significantly in the event of concomitant health disabilities.

Native American elderly.   Although the number of Native Americans dwelling on reservations declines, Native American peoples and their cultures persist. The high prevalence of alcoholism and its sequelae in some communities, early deterioration in physical health, and intergenerational distancing are particular problems for this population. Native theories of disease and herbal healing and the use of native healers are important to certain tribes. Although diagnostic criteria for depression and other mental illnesses must be studied further, the incidence of these disorders may not differ significantly from the incidence among non-Native Americans. Race or ethnicity-based differences in the risk of physical and mental illness, in the prevalence of particular diagnoses, and in sensitivity to medications have been suggested, but more definitive studies are needed to confirm their existence.

Current Recommendations

Additional reliable data are needed on the health and mental health needs of the minority elderly. National data sets and federally funded epidemiologic studies should oversample minority elderly to achieve statistically significant numbers to ensure development of reliable and valid analysis. Special areas of research focus should include the following:

✦ Establishing the prevalence and incidence of psychiatric disorders in ethnic minority elderly populations
✦ Evaluating the extent of misdiagnosis in ethnic minority elderly populations
✦ Validating clinical research instruments for studies of ethnic minority elderly populations
✦ Modifying existing instruments and developing new instruments to achieve more accurate diagnoses
✦ Encouraging program evaluation and development of model programs
✦ Evaluating alternative therapy approaches
✦ Conducting health services and policy research that will apply to ethnic minority elderly populations
✦ Evaluating the efficacy of existing treatments for minority elderly populations and establishing special guidelines, as needed, for medication use by, or psychotherapy with, these populations

Commitment for the Future

Because the deliberation of the task force illuminated issues for ongoing study, the APA has established a standing committee on minority elderly, under the purview of the Council on Aging within the APA, to do the following:

✦ Provide a focal point for the evaluation and study of the psychiatric problems of older immigrant, native, and bilingual populations
✦ Develop curriculum guidelines to sensitize medical students and general psychiatric residents to diagnostic and treatment issues of minority elderly individuals (in consultation with the APA Council on Medical Education)
✦ Disseminate approved curricular materials through special workshops at the APA annual meeting and appropriate publications
✦ Collect and disseminate information about model mental health programs for minority elderly to interested APA members and others

✦ Explore the controversy of mainstream versus segregated programs that specialize in cultural sensitivity.

✦ Work with the APA Division of Government Relations to develop policy recommendations for the improvement of funding and training opportunities in areas related to the mental health of the ethnic minority elderly and for the creation of special service-delivery provisions under Medicare and Medicaid

✦ Work with the APA Minority Researcher Training Program to encourage ethnic minority professionals to pursue research careers and to maintain an interest in research in minority issues

✦ Establish liaison with the minority committees from the Council on National Affairs and other relevant APA components

✦ Establish formal liaison with the Gerontological Society of America's Minority Elderly Committee; Alcohol, Drug Abuse, and Mental Health Administration (ADAMHA) institutes; and major ethnic minority advocacy groups

The task force has recommended that the APA support the following goals:

✦ Work to have government agencies and Congress mandate that appropriate minority sample size be achieved through oversampling in all national data sets to address questions about ethnic elderly

✦ Authorize the preparation of specific reports on minority elderly populations from the National Nursing Home Survey, Vital Statistics of the United States, and epidemiologic surveys supported by ADAMHA institutes

✦ Encourage Congress to fund demonstration projects of new, or replication of successful, mental health model programs for the ethnic minority elderly

✦ Encourage Congress to mandate the Health Care Financing Administration to develop specific funding for special programs for the highest-risk minority elderly populations (e.g., immigrants and Native Americans)

✦ Work for full Medicare and Medicaid eligibility for all seniors, irrespective of work history and residency status

✦ Encourage clinical training programs to remove bias against international medical graduates and to establish special training for bilingual individuals who want to enter psychiatry and work with their ethnic groups. There is still a bias against admitting international medical graduates or minority medical school residents in many training programs and difficulty capitalizing on the cultural identity of minority psychiatrists.

Chapter 2

National Data Bases on Minority Elders

James W. Thompson, M.D., M.P.H.

No extant national data bases provide information specifically on the psychiatric problems of minority elders. Even when data have been collected specifically on the minority elderly, samples rarely are of sufficient size to enable meaningful analysis. Thus, when analyzing data from existing national data sets, compromises must be made—either combining psychiatric diagnoses, whether severe or mild, or combining minority groups themselves. Neither compromise represents an acceptable approach that will help us understand the psychiatric needs of these diverse and growing populations.

Further, validity questions arise from the diversity of minority populations in our nation. Even in such large investigations as the Epidemiologic Catchment Area (ECA) program studies, minorities are often represented by only one or two subgroups from whom generalization becomes impossible. (For example, the "Hispanic" sample for the ECA studies comprised only Mexican Americans from a single ECA site.) For Native Americans and Asians, no cases were reported in the ECA data, highlighting the need for special sampling for groups that are small or geographically isolated. Undertaking large studies on even a small number of such subgroups is prohibitive; innovative methodologies must be devised to enable researchers to sample ethnic minorities in sufficient numbers to allow findings to be generalizable.

Even within the national population of the "elderly," it is difficult to make generalizations. There are great differences between the "old" (ages 65–84) and the "old-old" (ages 85 and over). Among minority population studies, definitions of age often differ from the norm. The age of 55, not 65, may be used as the lower boundary for an aged minority population. This "young-old" group may be very different from other minority elders.

Following are descriptions of two relevant epidemiologic studies that have included the elderly in their respective ethnic minority populations. Other data bases with some relevance to psychiatric disorders cover more of the demographic and social aspects of aging in minorities. Indeed, the task force literature review has highlighted the sad absence of data on psychiatric morbidity and treatment, and the task force emphasizes the need for collection of such data.

Epidemiologic Catchment Area Studies[1]

The ECA surveys were a series of National Institute of Mental Health (NIMH)–sponsored, community-based epidemiologic studies conducted in the early 1980s. The cities of New Haven, Connecticut; Baltimore, Maryland; St. Louis, Missouri; Durham, North Carolina (and surrounding counties); and Los Angeles, California, provided a randomly selected sample of households. The elderly were oversampled in New Haven and Baltimore using both the lay-administered Diagnostic Interview Schedule, from which DSM-III diagnoses could be simulated, and a services questionnaire designed for the study. There were over 18,000 unweighted subjects in the study. Although organic mental disorder was not included per se, it is approximated by "cognitive impairment," derived from the 20-item Mini-Mental State Exam.

The ECA data presented here are based, in some instances, on very few cases. Unlike other studies (including a recent review of anxiety disorders

[1]Thanks are due to Ann Hohmann, Sc.D., and Don Rae of the National Institute of Mental Health for consultation in analyzing the ECA data.

in the elderly from the Piedmont ECA study), the task force has not provided estimates of standard errors; rather, it has chosen not to report data based on fewer than 20 unweighted cases. The task force believes this to be necessary because, in the past, the minimal data available on these groups have been taken as definitive, even though investigators reporting such data have been careful to point out that the figures are based on very few cases. Even the data reported below should be used only for illustrative purposes, unless standard errors are estimated.

Table 2–1 shows a breakdown of the total ECA sample population by age, sex, and race. Table 2–2 shows the 6-month prevalence of disorders across sites by race for subjects between ages 18 and 54 and for subjects over age 54. Only whites, African Americans, and Hispanic Americans provide sufficient cases for analysis. Although subjects were chosen randomly within the ECA sites, the selection of sites was not random, per se. Therefore, these figures, particularly with regard to minorities, cannot be construed to be representative of the United States as a whole. Table 2–3 shows the presence of any diagnosis in the 6-month period by site. Again, in all tables except Table 2–1, which is simply the sample population

Table 2–1. Percentage of men and women in different age categories within races

Sex and age category	White	African American	Hispanic
Men			
< 55	70.1	79.9	84.9
55–64	15.3	10.3	8.5
65–74	9.6	6.7	4.3
75–84	4.2	2.6	2.0[a]
> 84	0.8	0.4[a]	0.4[a]
Women			
< 55	64.4	77.7	80.0
55–64	15.6	10.5	9.6
65–74	12.1	7.4	6.2
75–84	6.3	3.6	3.7
> 84	1.7	0.9	0.5[a]

Note. Data from Epidemiologic Catchment Area study. All sites included. Weighted.
[a]Based on fewer than 20 subjects.

Table 2–2. Percentage of psychiatric diagnoses in each race for ages 18–54

Diagnosis	Age group	White	African American	Hispanic
Bipolar[a]	18–54	1.1	1.3	—
	≥ 54	—	—	—
Major depression	18–54	4.4	3.7	4.2
	≥ 54	1.5	1.6	—
Dysthymia[a]	18–54	3.7	2.8	4.0
	≥ 54	2.5	1.8	—
Alcohol abuse	18–54	7.5	6.3	8.81
	≥ 54	2.1	3.3	—
Drug abuse	18–54	3.3	3.6	2.5
	≥ 54	—	0	0
Schizophrenia	18–54	1.1	1.8	—
	≥ 54	—	—	—
Schizophreniform	18–54	—	—	—
	≥ 54	0	0	0
Obsessive-compulsive	18–54	2.1	1.6	—
	≥ 54	0.9	1.9	0
Phobia	18–54	8.9	15.0	8.1
	≥ 54	6.7	13.9	9.1
Somatization	18–54	0	0	0
	≥ 54	0	0	0
Panic	18–54	1.2	1.2	—
	≥ 54	—	—	—
Antisocial personality[a]	18–54	1.6	1.2	—
	≥ 54	—	—	0
Cognitive impairment[b]	18–54	0.3	1.4	—
	≥ 54	2.3	9.2	—
Any DIS/DSM-III diagnosis	18–54	23.6	27.3	23.1
	≥ 54	14.0	24.7	18.5

Note. Data from Epidemiologic Catchment Area study. Six-month period. All sites included. Weighted. A dash indicates fewer than 20 unweighted positive cases. DIS = Diagnostic Interview Schedule.
[a]Lifetime diagnosis.
[b]Determined by Mini-Mental State Exam on day of interview.

Table 2–3.　Percentage of diagnoses at ECA sites for each race

ECA site	White	African American	Hispanic
New Haven, CT	19.5	21.8	35.8[a]
Baltimore, MD	24.2	31.8	—
St. Louis, MO	18.5	21.8	—
Durham, NC	22.1	29.4	—
Los Angeles, CA	20.5	20.7[b]	21.5

Note. All ages included. Weighted. A dash indicates fewer than 20 unweighted positive cases. ECA = Epidemiologic Catchment Area study.
[a]Fewer than 24 positive cases and of questionable use.
[b]Fewer than 33 positive cases and of questionable use.

breakdown, figures have been omitted when they are based on very few cases.

National Nursing Home Survey Pretest [2]

The National Nursing Home Survey pretest, sponsored in 1984 by the National Center for Health Statistics (NCHS) and NIMH, was conducted in a sample of skilled and intermediate nursing homes in four metropolitan areas: Atlanta, Georgia; Boston, Massachusetts; Denver, Colorado; and Toledo, Ohio. A stratified random sample of 150 homes was selected by bed size and type of facility ownership. Data were collected on 526 patients by trained interviewers, who conducted a structured interview with a staff nurse and examined each patient's medical records. Patients ages 65 and older were surveyed. (Only the data from this pretest are available, because NCHS elected not to include these psychiatric measures in the survey.)

Table 2–4 shows the percentage of both senile dementia/organic brain syndrome and other (nonorganic) mental disorders for different age categories. Again, only the white, African American, and Hispanic American

---

[2]Thanks to Penny Foval, Ph.D., formerly of the University of Maryland at Baltimore, for providing these data.

samples were large enough to report. The sites and nursing homes in the study were not chosen to be either representative of the United States or reflective of community rates.

Other Sources of Research Data

The National Archive of Computerized Data on Aging (NACDA) has a number of computerized data bases that are available for secondary analysis. The service operates under the auspices of the Inter-University Consortium for Political and Social Research (ICPSR). Most of the data bases address problem areas other than mental health and have significant limitations in use in the areas of mental health of the elderly and, more specifically, mental health of the minority elderly. Most researchers involved in the use of these data sets believe the quality of data and the data

Table 2–4.   Percentage of NNHS patients in age and diagnostic categories for each race

Diagnosis	White	African American	Hispanic
Ages 50–64			
Senile dementia/OBS	19.14	15.78	5.26
Other mental disorder	60.99	39.34	49.15
No mental disorder	19.87	44.88	45.59
Ages 65–74			
Senile dementia/OBS	32.58	44.50	50.52
Other mental disorder	34.37	28.96	28.80
No mental disorder	33.05	26.65	20.68
Ages 75–84			
Senile dementia/OBS	45.65	43.36	57.42
Other mental disorder	19.39	9.39	18.42
No mental disorder	34.96	47.25	24.16
Ages 85 and older			
Senile dementia/OBS	51.94	67.26	70.20
Other mental disorder	10.72	5.41	2.70
No mental disorder	37.34	27.33	27.10

Note.   NNHS = National Nursing Home Survey pretest, 1984. Weighted. OBS = organic brain syndrome.

items regarding mental health are limited. These data sets have not been analyzed specifically for questions about mental health concerns.

The most relevant data bases from NACDA for studies on mental health and health issues of minority elderly populations (obtained since 1980) are the following:

✦ Hispanic Health and Nutrition Examination Survey (HHANES), 1982–1984 (ICPSR #8535), contains questions on mental health and over-sampled the elderly

✦ Mexican origin people in the U.S.: The 1979 Chicano Survey (ICPSR #8436)

✦ Immigrants admitted to the U.S., 1988 (and annually, since 1972; ICPSR #8952–8966 and 9266–9269)

✦ The National Survey of Black Americans, 1979–1980 (ICPSR #8512)

✦ Americans' Changing Lives: Wave I, 1986 (ICPSR #9267), contains an oversampling of African Americans ($N = 1,131$) and individuals over age 60 ($N = 1,474$)

✦ National Health Interview Survey: Longitudinal Study of Aging (LSOA), 70 years and over, 1984–1987 (ICPSR #8719) contains data from Medicare Parts A and B and matches with the National Death Index; the study is ongoing

Conclusion

Nationally representative data on the minority elderly are sorely lacking. They can be obtained only by undertaking large stratified-sample studies within each minority population group. Too often, data about minorities based on only a few unrepresentative cases are quoted as definitive. The time has come to stop relying on such data and to examine scientifically the actual types and rates of mental disorder in the minority elderly.

Chapter 3

Issues in the Psychiatric Care of African American Elders

F. M. Baker, M.D., M.P.H.

Mr. J, a 62-year-old, childless, widowed African American, was referred for psychiatric evaluation during an inpatient medical admission. He had retired from the Postal Service to care for his wife of 40 years, who died of breast cancer 12 months prior to his hospitalization. He was referred for psychiatric evaluation because of increasing irascibility and irritability, coupled with a delusional belief that his roommate and the medical staff were spying on him and listening to his conversations. He was admitted for the management of congestive heart failure due to hypertension and arteriosclerotic heart disease. His family had noticed behavioral changes following his wife's death, which were continuing to worsen as his medical condition improved. His social support network consisted of a brother, a niece, and members of his church, where he served as an elder. His niece reported a history suggestive of bipolar II disorder with hypomania. He had two prior episodes of major depression, and one earlier episode of alcoholic hallucinosis misdiagnosed as paranoid schizophrenia. He was started on lithium and did well; 3 weeks later, he developed acute delirium due to lithium toxicity. He was found to be in acute renal failure. Hemoglobin electrophoresis showed hemoglobin S and hemoglobin C; his renal impairment seemed to be related to sludging of sickled red cells. After resolution of his toxic delirium, recovery of his renal status, and restabilization on a lower dose of lithium, Mr. J agreed to return for psychiatric care only at 6-month intervals "to help" his family practice

doctor. After 18 months, the lithium was discontinued. Mr. Jones has had
no relapse in a 3-year follow-up. He remains active in church, visits the
sick, and attends a group for widows and widowers.

Introduction

African Americans are a heterogeneous population of individuals with
"black" skin ranging in hue from café au lait to blue-black. In American
society, they represent one of several "visible minorities" who, in some
way, are physically different from Northern Europeans. Cultural values of
the various African tribal communities that emphasized collectivity, sharing, affiliation, obedience to authority, belief in spirituality, the importance
of the past, and respect for the elderly have been transmitted across generations, surviving the disruptions resulting from forced migration to the
Americas to become slaves.

Black individuals in the United States today include African Americans, African Caribbeans, and individuals of mixed ethnic heritage that
includes Northern European and American Indian components. Thus, the
United States black community encompasses a great diversity of cultures,
customs, languages, educational levels, and socioeconomic statuses.

According to the 1990 census, African Americans constitute 12% of
the United States population—almost 30 million individuals; 11.6% of the
total African American population are age 60 and older—3.4 million individuals. Individuals over age 85, the so-called "old-old," represent the
fastest-growing segment of the African American population. Whereas
10.7% of white Americans are classified as having incomes below the
poverty line, nearly 32% of African Americans fall below this line. A greater
percentage of African American elders than white American elders live
below the poverty line. Despite the income disparity, the average size of the
African family is slightly larger (3.4 members) than that of white American
families (3.11 members).

Census data in 1990 also show women representing 52.7% of the
African American population, 48.9% of whom were in the child-bearing
years (15–45 years). By age 30, the ratio of African American women to
men has reversed, so the number of women begins to exceed the number
of men. By late life, the number of women far exceeds that of men. The

greater longevity of African American women is due in large part to the early deaths of African American men (ages 18–28) by homicide, suicide, accidents, and substance abuse. Thus, African American elders are more likely to be older women of limited economic resources (United States Bureau of the Census 1992).

Almost all research has focused on the African American elder who grew up in the southern United States and migrated throughout the continental United States in the early 1900s. The increasing immigration of individuals of African heritage from the Caribbean islands, however, will contribute to the changing profile of the black population in the United States over at least the next 30 years. As immigrant African Caribbeans (formerly referred to as "West Indians") age, first-generation issues such as acculturation and language barriers will arise. Existing literature on African Caribbeans, though sparse, is included in the following bibliographic review.

The health of African Americans has been poorer than that of white Americans, whether measured by rates of infant mortality; prevalence of preventable diseases such as hypertension, obesity, and tuberculosis; or access to and use of health care resources. The Secretary's Task Force on Black and Minority Health documented the disparity in health status between ethnic minorities and whites in its six-volume report.

Background Bibliography

Baker FM, Lightfoot OB: Psychiatric care of ethnic elders, in Culture, Ethnicity, and Mental Illness. Edited by Gaw AC. Washington, DC, American Psychiatric Press, 1993, pp 517–552

Emphasizing the biopsychosocial model—understanding the interaction of biological factors and psychological health and the influence of the elders' social network in the development of disorder—the authors address the diversity of definitions of illness, loci of treatment, and expectations of Western medicine. A case example is presented for each of the four groups of ethnic elders: African American, American Indian and Alaska Native, Asian American, and Hispanic American. Specific lessons to be learned concerning the diagnosis, treatment, and management of psychiatric disorders in these ethnic elders are underscored. The chapter conclusion emphasizes the need to overcome the adversity of legalized segregation, exclusive legislation, and economic hardships for the majority of this cohort of ethnic elders. Literature regarding each group is cited to facilitate the reader's interest in expanding his or her knowledge base concerning a specific group.

Baker FM: Black youth suicide: literature review with a focus on prevention, in Report of the Secretary's Task Force on Youth Suicide, Vol 3: Prevention and Intervention in Youth Suicide (DHHS Publ No ADM-89-1623). Edited by Feinleib MR. Washington, DC, Alcohol, Drug Abuse, and Mental Health Administration, 1989, pp 177–195

The national rates of completed suicide in the African American population between 1950 and 1981 for ages 15–85 and older are presented, including age-adjusted rates. Specific studies of African American suicide attempters and completed suicide by African Americans in several cities (e.g., New York City; Philadelphia; Rochester, New York; New Haven, Connecticut) are discussed. Methodological problems with existing studies and national suicide statistics are presented. Proposed theories of African American suicide are reviewed. The article summarizes the literature on the characteristics of African American suicide attempters and presents specific preventive strategies at the primary, secondary, and tertiary levels of care.

Griffith EEH, Bell CC: Recent trends in suicide and homicide among blacks. JAMA 262:2265–2269, 1989

Suicide and homicide in the African American community are reviewed. The loss of African American men due to suicide and homicide, particularly among those ages 25–33, are noted as a major public health problem. The public health problems in the African American community are reviewed, approaches for attacking these problems are presented, and areas for future research are identified. Of particular note is the finding, based on data from the National Center for Health Statistics, that the rates of completed suicide among African American men ages 65 and older increased between 1970 and 1986. The authors suggest that this finding requires further investigation.

Manuel RC: The demography of older blacks in the United States, in The
  Black Elderly: Research on Physical and Psychosocial Health. Edited by
  Jackson JS. New York, Springer, 1988, pp 25–49

The author presents data to underscore his point that substantial
variation continues to exist in older populations. These variations are
important because they have implications for conclusions about the
level and nature of the needs of the older population, and for directions in research on the factors producing the unique patterns of the
data. Following a discussion of the growth and distribution of the older
African American or minority population and the older white population, several health-related indicators are analyzed, and income circumstances are detailed. The author provides a historical context by
discussing data from 1960 on, showing trends since the implementation of the domestic assistance programs of the Great Society legislation in the 1960s.

Gibson RC: Blacks in an Aging Society. New York, Carnegie Corporation,
  1986

This monograph is the outgrowth of a conference sponsored by the
Aging Society Project of the Carnegie Corporation of New York.
Twenty experts from a variety of disciplines met in October 1984 to
address the effects that the aging of American society and the evolving
fierce competition for available economic and social resources would
have upon the African American elderly. The monograph provides an
excellent summary of evolving trends affecting the social, economic,
physical, and psychological spheres of the aging African American
population. Pertinent data on longevity for whites and African Americans are presented. The implications of these data for the African
American elder and the multigenerational family are presented by the
participating experts. The monograph concludes with a discussion of
the importance of a life-span orientation to research. This approach
will allow the identification of cohort, period, and aging effects, either
longitudinally or by replicative cross-sectional data. These data will
provide information about changes in groups, individuals, and society
over time.

Task Force on Black and Minority Health: Report on Black and Minority Health, Vols 1–7. Washington, DC, Department of Health and Human Services, 1985

When the Secretary of Health and Human Services, Margaret Heckler, became aware of the disparity between African American and white Americans in infant mortality and homicide, she established a Task Force on Black and Minority Health to review the existing literature and data from national surveys to characterize the health of African Americans and other ethnic populations in comparison to white Americans. These publications detail the higher number of deaths for African Americans in various areas and discuss the implications. The data provide the most recent documentation of the disparity between different segments of the United States population along various health parameters.

Pinderhughes E: Afro-American families and the victim system, in Ethnicity and Family Therapy. Edited by McGoldrick M, Pearce JK, Giordano J. New York, Guilford, 1982, pp 108–122

The "victim system," created by barriers to opportunity and education, is explained as a circular feedback loop in which limited opportunities for achievement strain families, create suspiciousness and negative feelings, threaten self-esteem, and do not teach key skills. This system reinforces aberrant responses in communities, families, and individuals. Although elders are not specifically addressed, the chapter provides a context for intergenerational stresses and conflicts.

United States Bureau of the Census: Demographic aspects of aging and older populations in the United States, in Current Populations Reports: Special Studies. Washington, DC, U.S. Government Printing Office, 1980

Following an overview of the demographic characteristics of individuals ages 60 and older in 1980, specific tables of detailed information on education, residence, source of income, and several other variables are presented.

Wylie FM: Attitudes toward aging black Americans: some historical perspectives. Aging and Human Development 2:66–70, 1971

Reviewing the African cultural values that emphasized the worship of one's ancestors, the author traces these values to current African American families. The unique role of the older African American in his or her family is presented with an emphasis on the positive mental health benefits (definition of role and maintenance of a positive self-esteem). The author notes that from the West African cultural context, issues of "belongingness" rather than productivity appear to be dominant for African American elders.

Diagnostic Differences

Several authors have documented the particularly pernicious problem of misdiagnosis of psychiatric disorders in African American patients. Such patients are more likely to be diagnosed with schizophrenia, even when meeting diagnostic criteria for major affective disorders. Alcoholic hallucinosis, too, is often misdiagnosed as schizophrenic psychosis. Before the 1983 Epidemiologic Catchment Area (ECA) survey, few studies attempted to identify the prevalence of the major psychiatric disorders in African American populations. Only the National Survey of Black Americans interviewed a probability sample of community-resident African Americans. Although the National Black Survey provided significant information on social networks and perceptions of health, it was not designed to assess mental health or mental illness. Pooled data from the five U.S. cities participating in the ECA survey are shown in Tables 2–1 through 2–4 (see Chapter 2) but cannot be taken to be representative of the United States as a whole. Definitive studies of large stratified samples are needed to determine the specific prevalence of psychiatric disorders in African American elders.

The literature suggests that the types and rates of dementia in African American elders may differ from those of other racial groups. Black elderly individuals, for example, may be more prone to multi-infarct and alcoholic dementias due to the prevalence of obesity, diabetes, and hypertension. The rates of Alzheimer's disease appear to be the same for African Americans and whites based upon the few existing published studies. One population-based study in rural Mississippi found that African American elders ages 75 and older had higher rates of severe cognitive impairment than the older whites in this same county. The ECA study data from eastern Baltimore showed higher rates of multi-infarct dementia in those African American elders who had screened positive for cognitive impairment and who had completed a detailed evaluation for the etiology of their cognitive impairment.

The high prevalence of hypertension, cardiovascular disease, and diabetes increases the risks in African American elders for other dementias and episodes of delirium or organic mental syndromes. Studies have determined that the prevalence of hypertension among African American elders is higher than in the general population, but it is not clear whether the prevalence of multi-infarct dementia in African American elders is higher than the prevalence of clinically diagnosed Alzheimer's disease. Although the pattern of alcohol abuse in African Americans has been studied, the prevalence of alcohol dependence and alcoholic dementia remain unstudied in this population. It is not known, for instance, whether a reported pattern of earlier and heavier drinking in alcohol-abusing African Americans results in long-term cognitive deficits that manifest as alcoholic dementia or mixed dementia. Because multi-infarct dementia and alcoholic dementia are preventable dementias, further study in this area has profound implications for public policy, education, and health economics.

Existing instruments used to screen for cognitive impairment and depression may not "capture" all elderly African Americans affected by these disorders, because differences in communication style and educational level are still prevalent in this cohort of elders. Further validation and correction of these instruments, critical to ensuring their efficacy in identifying disorders in African American elderly individuals, is sorely needed. Such research should be undertaken by teams aware of and sensitive to the cultural concerns of African American elders. Further, such studies should include samples of both rural and urban elders in order to determine variance in the types of psychiatric disorders presenting in different settings. Although some investigators have questioned the validity of DSM-III-R diagnostic categories for the African American population, DSM-III-R is the current accepted standard for psychiatric diagnosis. If studies are to be comparable with the existing literature, research should rely on DSM-III-R diagnoses or on other widely accepted criteria as found in the Schedule for Affective Disorders and Schizophrenia or the Research Diagnostic Criteria.

Diagnostic Differences Bibliography

Baker FM: Dementing illness in African American populations: evaluation and management for the primary physician. J Geriatr Psychiatry 24(1):73–91, 1991

The author reviews international studies of dementing illness that report on prevalence of these disorders in various community populations in the United States, England, Finland, Sweden, Japan, and Italy. Two published studies from the United States contain significant numbers of African American elders. The data suggest that multi-infarct dementia has a higher prevalence in older African Americans than in other populations. Data from the National Health and Nutrition Examination Survey (NHANES) and the Secretary's Task Force on Black and Minority Health suggest that multi-infarct dementia and alcoholic dementia may be higher in the current population of African American elders compared with the cohort of white elders. These data are important, because the dementias to which they refer are all preventable. A discussion and case examples that differentiate between depression and dementia in African American elders are presented.

Baker FM: Afro-Americans, in Clinical Guidelines in Cross Cultural Mental Health. Edited by Comas-Dias L, Griffith EEH. New York, Wiley, 1988, pp 151–181

The author presents a historical overview of the diversity of the African American population in the United States. Following a discussion of demographic data, the African American family, and issues in clinical practice, the author discusses treatment issues across all age cohorts. She raises specific questions about the risk for alcoholic dementia in older African Americans. The paucity of data on psychiatric disorders in older African American elders is noted. The author suggests a secondary analysis of national data sets, such as the Epidemiologic Catchment Area survey, to tease out relevant data on African Americans from these existing samples.

Jackson JS: Growing old in black America: research on aging black populations, in The Black American Elderly: Research on Physical and Psychosocial Health. Edited by Jackson JJ. New York, Springer, 1988, pp 3–16

The author reviews the existing studies that comment on the characteristics of older African American individuals: the heterogeneity of this population, the increased survival of the "old-old," and issues of morbidity and mortality across the life cycle. Data on the specific health concerns of African American elders are presented as are specific data on the major causes of death. Specific information is presented on the four major sections of this text: demography and epidemiology of older African American adults, biological and health status, social and behavioral processes, and methodological issues in research on older African American adults.

Bell CC, Thompson JP, Lewis D, et al: Misdiagnosis of alcohol related organic brain syndromes: implications for treatment, in Treatment of Black Alcoholics. Edited by Brisbane FL, Womble M. New York, Haworth, 1985, pp 45–65

The authors present historical evidence that African American patients with organic brain syndromes (OBS) associated with alcoholism are often diagnosed as suffering from schizophrenia. Case histories of patients with alcohol-related OBS who have been diagnosed with schizophrenia are presented. The authors discuss the factors responsible for the misdiagnosis of African Americans with OBS associated with alcoholism. Treatment implications of misdiagnosis that results in inappropriate treatment with neuroleptics suggest a poor outcome for the African American alcoholic patient.

Schoenberg BS, Anderson DW, Harer AF: Severe dementia: prevalence and clinical features in a biracial U.S. population. Arch Neurol 42:740–743, 1985

Clinically diagnosed severe senile dementia of the Alzheimer's type was found at least as often among African Americans as among whites suffering from severe dementia. Among individuals 80 years of age or older, the prevalence for African Americans was 7% higher than for whites.

Jackson JS, Chatters L, Neighbors HW: The mental health status of older black Americans: a national study. Black Scholar 13:21–35, 1982

The authors present data on the mental health status of a large national sample of the African American elderly. Previous studies of mental health and illness in this population had been either geographically limited or based on small national samples that had not permitted reasonable investigation of important demographic differences. In addition to traditional measures of self-reported mental health functioning, this study also includes measures of well-being in an attempt to explore the multidimensional nature of the mental health concept in the African American elderly. The authors find a great deal of heterogeneity among the African American elderly, and significant relationships between global measures of well-being and measures of psychological distress. The implications of these findings for a multidimensional concept of mental health in African Americans are discussed.

Adebimpe VR: Hallucinations and delusions in black psychiatric patients. J Natl Med Assoc 73:517–520, 1981

Using observational data, the author confirms the hypothesis of a higher incidence of hallucinations reported among African American patients than among white patients with schizophrenia. African Americans, irrespective of diagnosis, experience a variety of nonschizophrenic hallucinations. The authors suggest that lack of familiarity with the content of hallucinations in African Americans has led to erroneous diagnoses of schizophrenia.

Jones BE, Gray BA, Parson EB: Manic-depressive illness among poor urban blacks. Am J Psychiatry 1185:654–657, 1981

A sample of 117 African American psychiatric patients was examined to assess manic-depressive disorder and socioeconomic characteristics. Approximately 15% of the sample who actually carried other chart diagnoses were found to suffer from manic-depressive illness. The authors explain the ramifications of misdiagnosis and the need for future investigations.

Bell C, Mehte H: The misdiagnosis of black patients with manic-depressive illness. J Natl Med Assoc 72:141–145, 1979

Three case histories highlight the authors' contention that African American patients with manic-depressive disorder are frequently misdiagnosed as having chronic undifferentiated schizophrenia and treated with major tranquilizers without the initiation of a mood stabilizing medication such as lithium or carbamazepine.

Helzer J: Bipolar affective disorders in black and white men. Arch Gen Psychiatry 32:1140–1143, 1975

The author analyzes demographic, clinical, and family history variables of 11 African American and 19 white men with diagnoses of manic-depressive disorder. With the exception of a greater preponderance of alcoholism in the paternal relatives of the African American men, the clinical and familial expression of bipolar affective disorder is similar in the two races.

Kramer M, Rosen M, Willis EM: Definition and distribution of mental disorders in a racist society, in Racism and Mental Health. Edited by Willie CV, Kramer BM, Brown BS. Pittsburgh, PA, University of Pittsburgh Press, 1973, pp 353–459

Detailed data from community studies undertaken to determine the prevalence of mental disorders in the United States are presented. Also, data on patterns of the use of psychiatric facilities by race are reviewed. The inadequacy of present statistics on mental disorders by race are discussed. Specific recommendations are made for the development of statistics that can serve as the basis of programs to eliminate the attitudes, practices, and conditions that adversely affect the physical and mental health of citizens of the United States.

Liss JL, Weiner A, Robins E, et al: Psychiatric symptoms in white and black inpatients. Compr Psychiatry 14:475–481, 1973

Differences in psychiatric symptomatology between African American and white groups were attributable to different frequencies of psychiatric disorders in these groups. The authors state that dull affect, delusions of grandeur, delusions of passivity, fighting, and auditory and visual hallucinations were significantly more frequent among the African American patients. Because selection factors prompting hospitalization were similar in both sample groups, differences in symptoms between African American and white patients could not be explained by a difference in frequency of psychiatric disorders. Moreover, the association of symptoms with specific psychiatric diagnoses was greater in the white than in the African American population.

Simon RJ, Fleiss JL, Gurland BJ, et al: Depression and schizophrenic hospitalized black and white mental patients. Arch Gen Psychiatry 28:509–512, 1973

The authors compare racial differences in diagnoses made by hospital-based psychiatrists and research psychiatrists. Hospitals were found to diagnose African Americans with schizophrenia rather than affective disorders more often than they diagnosed whites. When research psychiatrists applied the Research Diagnostic Criteria (RDC), race and diagnosis functioned independently. Black patients diagnosed by the RDC with affective disorder were diagnosed by the hospital psychiatrists as having schizophrenia. When depressive disorders were examined, the authors found that hallucinations and delusions in African American patients were diagnosed as schizophrenia.

Wilcox P: Positive mental health in the black community: the black liberation movement, in Racism and Mental Health. Edited by Willie CV, Kramer BK, Brown BS. Pittsburgh, PA, University of Pittsburgh Press, 1973, pp 463–482

In this chapter, the author addresses the concept of positive mental health from the African American perspective. The essential components of the black liberation movement of the 1960s are reviewed; the self-liberating activities that emerged in African American communities are discussed. Wilcox concludes with a discussion of the mental health implications of these activities.

Sletten J, Schuff S, Altman H, et al: A statewide computerized psychiatric system: demographic, diagnostic, and mental status data. Int J Soc Psychiatry 18:30–40, 1972

Relationships among demographic variables, mental status, and psychiatric diagnoses of 4,156 patients are described. Although the article does not focus on elderly African Americans, it does address a positive correlation in increased frequency of admissions in an older age group. Older patients are more likely to have signs of organic grandiose delusions and reduced speech noted on mental status examinations, and have different admission characteristics.

Cannon M, Locke BZ: Being black is detrimental to one's mental health: myth or reality? Phylon 38:408–428, 1967

The authors evaluate the mental health of African Americans. Using available data, they attempt to determine whether the gap in mental health status between African Americans and whites has been closing and to answer the question, "Is being African American detrimental to one's mental health?" Difficulties encountered included the absence of systematically collected mental health data on African Americans, the division of existing data into white and nonwhite categories only, and the inadequacy of definitions of mental health. Following an extensive review of mental health trends, patterns of admission and institutionalization, and a review of the locus of treatment and characteristics of therapists, the authors conclude that the amount of melanin in the skin is not related to mental disorders. In the authors' judgment, the stressful social conditions resulting from being African American, however, do contribute to the high prevalence of mental disorders among African Americans. Specific examples of stressful social conditions include experiences of loss or failure; denial of respect, dignity, and courtesy; treatment as inferior; and the effects of institutional racism. The importance of poverty secondary to racism in understanding the societal and socioeconomic reality for African Americans is emphasized.

Vitols MM, Water HG, Keeler MH: Hallucinations and delusions in white and Negro schizophrenics. Am J Psychiatry 120:472–476, 1963

This research found the incidence of hallucinations among African Americans with schizophrenia to be significantly higher than that found in whites with the same disorder. However, the incidence of delusions was found to be equal for both groups. The authors further posit that cultural patterns may be responsible for the difference in the rate of occurrence of hallucinations.

Health and Mortality Issues

Life expectancy at birth specifies the average number of years that an individual will live, going by the age-specific death rates prevailing in the year of his or her birth. The life expectancy for white Americans born in 1980 was 74.4 years; African Americans would be expected to live for 68 years. Although both men and women of all racial groups are living longer, life expectancy among African American men remains the lowest of all race-sex groups (see Table 3–1).

In 1980, 15 causes of death accounted for 89.1% of the total number of deaths for African Americans. In 13 of the 15 categories, African Americans experienced higher rates than white Americans (see Table 3–2). Only chronic obstructive pulmonary disease and suicide rates were lower in African Americans than in whites. The older African American is more likely than his or her white counterpart to suffer from chronic illness, with its associated morbidity and mortality. With less formal education (less than 8th grade), African American patients are more likely to screen falsely positive for cognitive impairment. Although rates of depression appear to be very high in medically ill patients, only scattered data from national data bases and the Secretary's Task Force on Black and Minority Health provide

Table 3–1. Life expectancy (years) for race-sex groupings in 1970 and 1980

Race-sex grouping	Life expectancy in 1970	Life expectancy in 1980	Change in life expectancy from 1970 to 1980
White women	75.6	78.1	+2.5
Black women	68.3	72.3	+4.0
White men	68.0	70.7	+2.7
Black men	60.0	63.7	+3.7

Table 3–2. Ratio of African American age-adjusted death rates (AADRs) to white AADRs for different causes of death

Cause of death	Ratio of African American to white AADRs	Comparison (men:women)
Heart disease	1.3:1	2:1
Malignant neoplasms, including neoplasms of lymphatic and hematopoeitic tissue	1.3:1	1.5:1
Cerebrovascular disease	1.8:1	1.2:1
Accidents and adverse effects, excluding motor vehicle accidents	1.8:1	3:1
Pneumonia and influenza	1.6:1	1.8:1
Diabetes mellitus	2.2:1	1:1[a]
Chronic liver disease and cirrhosis	2.0:1	2:1
Atherosclerosis	1.1:1	1.3:1
Homicide and legal interventions	5.9:1	3.9:1
Certain conditions originating in the perinatal period	2.0:1	NC
Nephritis, nephrotic syndrome, nephrosis	3.2:1	1.6:1
Congenital anomalies	3.2:1	NC
Septicemia	3.0:1	_____

Note. NC = no comparison.
[a]Only 2% greater.

insight into both medical illnesses and psychiatric disorders in African American elders.

African Americans who reach their sixth decade of life are unique. They have survived low birth weight and prematurity, the risk of death from homicide in their child and adolescent years, increased lifetime risk from accidents, and higher risks of cirrhosis, diabetes, cancer, and atherosclerosis due to patterns of early and high use of cigarettes, alcohol, and foods high in fat and low in fiber. Indeed, African Americans surviving to age 75 will live longer than white Americans of the same age. In 1978, an African American woman, age 80, had a life expectancy of 11.5 additional years whereas an 80-year-old white woman had a life expectancy of only 8.8 additional years. In 1978, an African American man, age 80, had a life expectancy of 8.8 more years; a white man of the same age had a life expectancy of only 6.7 more years. At younger ages, life expectancy for African Americans is significantly lower than for the white majority. This "crossover" effect, in which life expectancy of African American elders begins to exceed the white majority's life expectancy, requires further study.

Health and Mortality Issues Bibliography

Baker FM, Lavizzo-Mourey R, Jones BE: Acute care of the African American elder. J Geriatr Psychiatry Neurol (in press)

The provision of emergency psychiatric care to African American elders is discussed. Beginning with a review of the major health problems of African American elders and the pharmacologic treatment of these medical illnesses, the various types of psychiatric symptoms and psychiatric disorders that can be seen in a population of older African Americans are described. Specific strategies and concerns for the management of both physical and psychiatric illnesses are detailed. The article concludes with a consideration of the specific types of policy and programmatic initiatives required to plan a comprehensive system of psychiatric services for African American elders.

Drury TR, Powell AL: Prevalence of diabetes among black Americans, in Advance Data from Vital and Health Statistics, No 130 (DHHS Publ No

PHS-87-1250). Hyattsville, MD, National Center for Health Statistics, Public Health Service, 1989

Statistical data on the prevalence of diabetes in African Americans of various age cohorts is presented. Rates of diabetes are significantly higher for all age groups.

Baquet CR: Cancer prevention and control in the black population: epidemiology and aging implications, in The Black American Elderly: Research on Physical and Psychosocial Health. Edited by Jackson JS. New York, Springer, 1988, pp 50–68

Using data from the national Surveillance, Epidemiology, and End Results (SEER) program, the author examines the higher cancer incidence and mortality rates in the African American population. Although the African American population as a whole is younger than the white population, the data show that through their seventh decade of life, older African American individuals have higher rates of various cancers than whites. Specific points presented include 1) for all cancers combined, African American men have a higher rate than whites until age 75; 2) African American women have a higher age-specific incidence of breast cancer up to around age 40, when the incidence declines; 3) esophageal cancer rates for African American men and women are greater at all ages; 4) prostate cancer rates for African American men are higher at all age groups; 5) stomach cancer rates are higher in African Americans at all age groups for both sexes; and 6) 5-year relative survival was 12 percentage points lower for African Americans, with marked differences for cancers of the bladder, breast (women), uterus, prostate, and rectum. Baquet concludes with an overview of the risk factors and exposures that relate to the higher incidence rates for the African American population and addresses issues of cancer-related knowledge, attitudes, and practices in this population. Specific areas of needed research investigation are detailed.

Jackson JS: Survey research in aging black populations, in The Black American Elderly: Research on Physical and Psychological Health. Edited by Jackson JS. New York, Springer, 1988, pp 327–346

The author discusses the application of survey research methods in African American populations. He provides examples of the large number of poor survey studies conducted in the past, particularly problems in drawing adequate samples, designing appropriate instruments, coding, analysis, and interpretation. Attention is called to the importance of recognizing specific age cohort concerns; for example, older cohorts of African Americans born or reared in the South possess distinctive language patterns compared with whites and other African Americans that affect questionnaire design. Jackson concludes with a detailed discussion of the various response errors (sampling errors, nonresponse errors, task errors, interviewer errors, and respondent errors) and provides specific approaches to handling the problems in African American samples.

Presentation of Psychiatric Disorders

The presenting symptoms of psychiatric illness in African American populations have often been described as being "different" or "atypical." Confusion or psychotic symptoms such as hallucinations and delusions, for example, seem to occur with depression in African Americans. Presenting psychiatric symptoms in elderly African Americans are often blurred by the effects of socioeconomic status, chronic and untreated medical problems, and a history of inadequate or inappropriate treatment.

The legacy of segregated health care facilities, coupled with racism's effect on the locus of treatment, and the therapeutic interaction with professionals is part of the life experience of African American elders. Although African American elders' knowledge of psychiatric disorders has expanded as the result of increased media attention to mental illness, specialist treatment is rarely sought. The family physician who has earned the trust of the African American elder remains crucial to the identification, management, and treatment referral of African American elderly individuals suffering from psychiatric disorders.

In contrast to other ethnic minorities, most African Americans have no tradition of myths or cultural beliefs about mental illness. However, common terms used to describe mental illness include "going off," "having trouble," or "not right in the head." The impact of poverty, chronic physical illness, and, in central cities, the chronic stress of increased crime, may place some African American elders at increased risk for adjustment or anxiety disorders. Again, there are no studies that systematically assess these hypotheses.

Two studies assessing depressive illness in samples of ambulatory medical patients that include a significant percentage of African American patients found that one-third of the African American patients in these medical clinics had a diagnosis of major depressive disorder.

Presentation of Psychiatric Disorders Bibliography

Baker FM: The Afro-American life cycle: success, failure, and mental health. J Natl Med Assoc 79:625–633, 1987

The psychosocial context of the African American life cycle from the 1900s to the 1980s is examined through a case example of a three-generation African American family living in the United States in the 1980s. The article identifies the specific stresses and coping strategies of the family members and discusses the potential mental and emotional health problems arising from ineffective mastery of developmental transitions.

Brantley T: Racism and its impact on psychotherapy. Am J Psychiatry 140:1605–1608, 1983

The author expresses concern about the impact of racial issues on the therapeutic encounter, particularly when presenting problems relate to prejudice, discrimination, or both. The need for neutral therapeutic alliances across age boundaries is emphasized.

Carter JH: The black aged: implications for mental health care. J Am Geriatr Soc 30:67–70, 1982

Carter reviews the specific concerns of African American elders based on both a literature review and an African American psychiatrist's clinical experience. He describes the problems arising in the diagnosis of mental illness and the selection of services that result from both racism and the lack of sensitivity to racial and ethnic differences. Accounts of excessive use of physical restraints, questionable use of long-term electroconvulsive therapy and neuroleptics, and lack of informed consent suggest past inattention to the treatment needs of this population. The presence of African American health care providers and administrators results in increased use of services by African American elders. The author posits that to establish specific treatments for mental disorders among the African American aged, a practitioner must have in-depth knowledge of and sensitivity to their values, beliefs, and life-styles. The article also lists major resources for the African American elderly: the Center for Minority Group Mental Health Programs, the minority technical assistance services of the various regional mental health offices, and the National Caucus on the Black Aged.

Powell GJ: Overview of the epidemiology of mental illness among Afro-Americans, in The Afro-American Family: Assessment, Treatment, and Research Issues. Edited by Bass BA, Wyatt GE, Powell GJ. New York, Grune & Stratton, 1982, pp 155–163

The author reviews the limitations and methodological weaknesses of existing epidemiologic studies of mental disorders in the African American population. Beginning with definitions of society and culture, and discussion of Meyer's urban stress model, differences in mental illnesses between African American and white samples are presented, based on publications of the 1950s and 1960s. Problems in these studies relate to overgeneralizations about the African American population. Small sample size, the mixing of various disparate institutional settings, and diagnostic bias contributed to the difficulty in interpreting existing data. For example, Powell reports that in 1969, approximately one of every 100 nonwhite women between the ages of 35 and 45 was admitted to either a public mental hospital or an outpatient psychiatric clinic with a diagnosis of schizophrenia. The chapter concludes with a review of data from the President's Commission on Mental Health Subpanel on Afro-Americans. One conclusion of this subpanel was that the mental health of African Americans must be conceived within the context of "the total cultural and societal system," which includes people's feelings of self-worth within the societal system and within the identifiable group to which they belong.

Adebimpe VR: Overview: white norms and psychiatric diagnosis of black patients. Am J Psychiatry 138:279–285, 1981

Allegations of psychiatric misdiagnosis of African American patients are supported by only a few examples of such errors. However, a modest body of circumstantial evidence suggests that African American patients run a higher risk of being misdiagnosed than white patients. The author reviews the studies providing such evidence and concludes that greater awareness among clinicians and research into more appropriate diagnostic criteria for African American patients are desirable.

President's Commission on Mental Health: Reports of Special Populations Subpanel on Mental Health of Black Americans, Vol 2 Appendix. Washington, DC, U.S. Government Printing Office, 1978

The Subpanel on Mental Health of Black Americans reviewed the demographic and social characteristics of the population, discussed the existing knowledge of mental illness in this population, and reviewed the conflicting epidemiologic data. The impact of these data on diagnosis, rates of institutionalization, and patterns of treatment are discussed. The report concludes with a series of recommendations regarding mental health personnel, research directions, and the need to develop specific preventive strategies for the African American population.

Jackson JJ: The plight of older black women in the United States. Black Scholar 7:47–55, 1976

In 1970, 2.9 million African American women were age 45 and older; by 1994, that number will rise to 4.4 million. The specific plight of older African American women is presented in four key spheres: economics, relationships, mortality, and social networks.

Raskin A, Crook TH, Herman KD: Psychiatric history and symptom differences in black and white depressed inpatients. J Consult Clin Psychol 43:73–80, 1975

The authors compared 159 African American and 555 white depressed patients on social, personality, psychiatric history, and presenting symptoms while controlling for race differences, age, socioeconomic status, and sex. African Americans showed a greater tendency toward negativism and the introjection of anger. Depressed African American men were more likely to strike back verbally or physically when they perceived their rights were being violated. A much higher incidence of suicide threats or attempts was found among depressed African American men.

Jackson JJ: "Help me somebody! I's an old black standing in the need of institutionalizing." Psychiatric Opinion 10:6–16, 1973

Mortality data on African American elders (1970) showed a lower life expectancy for African American men; consequently, older women significantly outnumbered men. Further, the author found that the increased likelihood of urban residence—particularly in central cities—decreased access to care. In 1970, almost 61% of African Americans ages 65 or older were identified as living in the South. Fifty percent of African American elders lived in poverty. Poverty, place of residence, and limited access to mental health services or practitioners of similar background severely limited care for this population and increased stressors. The author notes that no systematic studies have been completed on the nature of service-use barriers encountered by African American elderly individuals. The article concludes with a summary of recommendations from the National Caucus on the Black Aged and the Special Concerns Session on Aging and Aged Blacks, 1971 White House Conference on Aging.

Pinderhughes CA: Racism and psychotherapy, in Racism and Mental Health. Edited by Willie CV, Kramer BM, Brown BS. Pittsburgh, PA, University of Pittsburgh Press, 1973, pp 61–121

The origins of racism and a history of racism in the United States are presented. A description of the psychotherapy of African Americans before and after 1967 is given with case histories. Social and psychological repression contribute to the need for psychotherapy. Biracial relationships in psychotherapy and racism in therapists are considered. This chapter concludes with a discussion of the patterns encountered in all repressive societies. Addressing the differences between societies based on competition and on sharing, the author presents 12 hypotheses concerning the interaction between repressing forces and the repressed in somatic, psychological, and social fields as well as discussing the implications of these hypotheses.

Carter JH: "Differential" treatment of the elderly black: victims of stereotyping. Postgrad Med 52:211–214, 1972

The author emphasizes the importance of cultural and social intervention within the framework of medical care for African American elderly individuals. The risks in stereotyping the elderly by physicians are described. Carter recommends that physicians seek special cultural education, including greater community involvement, to better understand the treatment needs of African American elderly.

Crawford FR: Variations between Negroes and whites in concepts of mental illness, its treatment, and prevalence, in Changing Perspectives in Mental Illness. Edited by Plog SS, Edgerton RB. New York, Holt, Rinehart & Winston, 1969, pp 242–256

This chapter appeared at the time of the civil rights movement of the 1960s. In this period, the reliability and validity of existing data on "Negro" Americans were questioned; studies assessing mental illness in African American and white populations were also questioned. This author emphasizes the lack of coordination in data collection—even in federally funded programs in all 50 states. Although case registers expanded patient data reporting systems and computerized analytic procedures, Crawford criticizes the data produced as largely uncoordinated and difficult to interpret and compare. The application of statistical techniques to assess the significance of, potential for error in, and confidence intervals for reported findings, in general, was not done. Crawford cites work of his group and others that found that African American patients continued to have little chance of receiving the full range of services available to whites. He notes that the African American population is heterogeneous in income, education, occupation, life goals; it is not monolithic. He calls for more careful research into the attitudes and values held by African Americans and whites at different socioeconomic levels and urges that a study be conducted examining the methods and definitions for determining a diagnosis of mental illness and evaluating differences in the care provided.

Special Areas of Concern

To understand the reactions and expectations of African Americans to the care systems available to them, it is important to understand the history of the subgroups and their cultural and geographical settings. Africans were forcibly removed from their agrarian or nomadic tribal communities that emphasized the value of family and the good of the community. Along with some other ethnic groups, Africans were used as slave labor, suffering deplorable hardship and mortality. Because slavery in the United States disrupted family bonds and community ties among individuals from several predominantly West African tribal groups with different languages and religions, alternative extended families evolved. The African American elder of the 1990s has heard the oral history of the dark passage, slavery, and reconstruction, and has experienced personally segregation, desegregation, the civil rights movement of the 1960s, as well as three major wars (World War II, the Korean War, and the Vietnam War).

The civil rights movement of the 1960s confronted institutional racism and emphasized the positive aspects of African American culture. Although the movement resulted in many new programs, today health care programs for most African Americans are still inadequate; many African Americans of all age groups still mistrust traditional service systems. The African American elder's skepticism of the American health care system is influenced by past experience in a segregated system in which physicians willing to treat "colored patients" were hard to find, and medications were too expensive to purchase. Historically excluded from mainstream health services, the African American learned to depend on indigenous healers who used the plants, roots, and native barks to make teas and poultices to "purge" the gastrointestinal system to prevent parasitic infections, to facilitate wound healing, and to alleviate fatigue and menstrual pain. Although today, with the access afforded by Medicare, most African American elders seek mainstream health care, they are more likely to be seen in a clinic rather than in a private physician's office. The African American elder retains some suspicion about the reception he or she will receive from health care providers.

Beginning in the 1970s, middle-class African American families started a reverse migration to the southern hometowns of their parents and grandparents to remove their children from the stresses, substance abuse problems, and poor educational systems of large urban cities. This may lead to new problems in service delivery for future cohorts of African American elders.

Special Areas of Concern Bibliography

Baker FM, Williams L, Bailey SF, et al: Black middle-class women in San Antonio, TX: coping strategies. J Natl Med Assoc 84(6):497–502, 1992

A significant portion of the literature on African Americans has focused on the lowest socioeconomic strata of this population. This study focuses on the identification of middle-class (as defined by the Hollingshead and Redlich Two-Factor Index of Social Position) African American women in San Antonio, Texas, in order to describe their education, work, marital status, and family size; the presence of medical and psychiatric illnesses; the significant events and individuals that influenced them; and the supportive resources they draw upon. When asked to make specific recommendations to African Americans and, specifically, to African American women, this convenience sample of 56 middle-class African American women emphasized striving to attain one's goal, doing one's best, developing self-esteem and self-love, the importance of education, the knowledge of African American history, and self-sacrifice and cooperation to target the serious problems affecting all African American people.

Coner-Edwards AF, Spurlock J: Black Families in Crisis: The Middle Class. New York, Brunner/Mazel, 1988

The various contributing authors address the characteristics, experiences, dynamics, accomplishments, and problems of African American families in the expanding African American middle class. Defining stress as a physical or psychological stimulus that produces strain or disequilibrium when impinging upon an individual, the editors observe that stresses weathered without any untoward or overt disorder may exact a psychological cost. Others experience mild, moderate or severe impairment. The editors note that the absence of stresses generated by poverty and poor educational opportunities do not necessarily make for immunity to mental illness in the middle class. This is one of the few published texts that address the economic diversity within the African American community and assess the unique perspectives of African American middle-class men and women.

Griffith EEH, Young JL, Smith DL: An analysis of the therapeutic elements in a black church service. Hosp Community Psychiatry 35:464–469, 1984

Twenty individuals who frequently attend a mid-week service at an independent African American church were interviewed by the authors to determine the nature of their experience during the service. Their replies suggested that the service as a whole imparted feelings of group closeness and strength akin to the curative factors associated with group psychotherapy. The results suggest that the African American church service is a functional community mental health resource for its participants.

Baker FM: The black elderly: biopsychosocial perspective within an age cohort and adult development context. J Geriatr Psychiatry 15:227–239, 1982

Recent literature is reviewed emphasizing the heterogeneity of the African American population, health outcomes for African Americans, and the historical experience of African American elders in the United

States. The macrohistorical context is related to the definition of illness and treatment expectations of one African American elderly woman in a hospital setting. Cultural problems of staff are also noted, such as potential misinterpretations of target behaviors.

Heisel MA, Faulkner A: Religiosity in an older black population. Gerontologist 22:354–358, 1982

A group of 122 urban African American respondents, 51–90 years of age, were interviewed about their religious practices and beliefs. The results were analyzed using a multidimensional scale based on Block's conceptual framework. Religiosity did not appear to vary with age, but church membership did. Women had higher scores than men; religiosity was positively related to life satisfaction and to frequency of church attendance regardless of age and sex.

Spurlock J: Black Americans, in Cross-Cultural Psychiatry. Edited by Gaw A. Boston, MA, John Wright, 1982, pp 163–178

The author establishes the context of American society and its negative media stereotyping of African Americans. Addressing the importance of developing culturally relevant curricula in psychiatric residency training programs, Spurlock reviews the myths about African American individuals in America. Following comments with pertinent references regarding effective psychiatric techniques, she concludes with three essentials for culturally relevant curricula: 1) recognition of the hazards of the "deficit model" and attention to the possible norms in differences; 2) a representative sample of African American–related references in assigned readings for literature seminars or other pertinent components of the training program; and 3) clinical experiences with patients from different cultural backgrounds than the trainee's should occur as should supervision by a faculty member of a different cultural background.

McAdoo H: Factors related to stability in upwardly mobile black families. Journal of Marriage and Family 40:761–776, 1978

The impact of upward mobility over three generations on the extended kin network of African American parents in the mid-Atlantic area was examined. Extensive involvement has been maintained by those born in both the middle and working classes and those living in urban and suburban sites. The reciprocal obligations of the help exchange patterns were not perceived as excessive, but were stronger for those born in the working class. Educational achievement and maternal employment peaked in the generation in which mobility occurred. Kin interaction was high with low geographic mobility. Results indicate that extended help patterns are culturally rather than economically based.

Martin EP, Marin JH: The Black Extended Family. Chicago, IL, University of Chicago Press, 1978

The authors present data from an 8-year study of 30 African American extended families including more than 1,000 individuals. The authors address such fundamental questions as: How is the African American extended family composed, and what are its functions? How do young and old, male and female, "better off" and "worse off," and rural and urban family members relate to one another? How is the extended family affected by social change, and what are its prospects for survival? This is one book in an emerging body of literature on the multigenerational, independent kinship system of the African American family that is welded together by a sense of obligation to relatives.

Dancy J Jr: The Black Elderly: A Guide for Practitioners with Comprehensive Bibliography. Ann Arbor, MI, The Institute of Gerontology at the University of Michigan–Wayne State University, 1977

This volume provides an overview of older individuals in the United States, presenting a profile of the African American elder: demographic data, family ties, religion, employment patterns, food preferences, language patterns, coping behaviors, and strengths. The monograph includes a highly detailed bibliography.

Gutman H: The Black Family in Slavery and Freedom. New York, Pantheon, 1976

This is one of the few books that follow the African American family and its composition from the period of Reconstruction to the present. Alternative patterns of family structure that have evolved are reviewed. The specific implications of this historical context are presented.

Family and Support Issues

The family serves as a particularly important means of support for African Americans with mental illness due, in part, to the history of segregation and institutional bias against hospital admissions for African Americans with psychiatric disorders. In the past, families tolerated unusual behavior and cared for the mentally ill at home unless they became violent. Although possible in the predominantly agrarian society of the early 1900s, tolerance of deviant or psychotic behavior in an urban central city, particularly in a one-room apartment in a housing project in the central city, became wholly unrealistic.

The mental health needs of African Americans are influenced by their socioeconomic status. Families above the poverty level function well with mutuality in leadership and involvement in a range of community activities. In contrast, families below the poverty level are so concerned with simple survival that families often become dysfunctional in reaction to these ongoing stresses. Family support for the mentally ill elderly, understandably, becomes difficult for a dysfunctional family.

Several authors emphasize that mental health and self-esteem among African American elders are strengthened by their roles within the African American extended family, the community, and the African American church. The lower suicide rates noted in older African American men and women, in part, have been attributed to the roles assumed by the elder. Retirement from gainful employment does not end the opportunity for mentorship and leadership by the African American elderly man as it may for his white counterpart.

The African American extended family remains an important source of financial and emotional support for the elder in the 1990s. Even if adult children reside in another city, they can mobilize the elder's support network of church or club members to provide daily contact with the elder. Supervision of medication regimens, provision of transportation, and meal preparation can be undertaken by this extended family network.

Family and Support Issues Bibliography

Lawson WB: Chronic mental illness and the black family. American Journal of Social Psychiatry 6:57–61, 1986

Having reviewed the historical literature relating abnormal patterns of communication to the incidence of schizophrenia, Lawson looks at African American families to assess the hypothesis that schizophrenia is caused by personal experience with family members. He reviews the recent literature on African American families and addresses the failure of the Moynihan report to recognize the effects of alternative family structures among African American families, the ongoing psychosocial pressures, the effects of slavery, and the consequences of poverty. The Moynihan report characterized the African American family as a tangle of pathology. The author attributed the problems of teenage pregnancy and substance abuse to single-parent families and especially African American women. Lawson reports studies that show that 50%–75% of the chronically mentally ill in the community live with their families. This fact has special significance for the families of African Americans and other minorities. In addition to the increased likelihood of a family being labeled pathological, a family is more susceptible to the negative consequences of having an ill member. The ongoing need to cope with racial discrimination, coupled with fewer economic resources, contributes to the increased susceptibility of the African American family caring for a member with a chronic mental illness. The author discusses the strengths of the African American family and describes alternatives to traditional family therapy.

Taylor R, Chatters LM: Patterns of informal support to elderly black adults: family, friends, and church members. Social Work 31:432–438, 1986

Patterns of concomitant support to elderly African Americans from family, friends, and church members were examined using the National Survey of Black Americans. Eight of 10 respondents reported receiving assistance from friends, 6 of 10 received aid from church members, and over half received support from families. Few respondents were defined as *socially isolated.*

Chatters LM, Taylor RJ, Jackson JS: Size and composition of the informal helper networks of elderly blacks. J Gerontol 40:605–614, 1985

Research on the informal support networks of older individuals recognizes that network size and composition have important consequences for care. Factors that determine the characteristics of networks of older African Americans, however, have not been explored systematically. The study examines the relationship of a group of sociodemographic, health, family, and availability factors to the size and composition of informal support networks. The data were taken from the National Survey of Black Americans and constitute a nationally representative sample ($N = 581$) of older African Americans, ages 55 and older. The results for several of the sociodemographic factors (e.g., sex and marital status) are consistent with previous work, and show regional differences. The findings underscore the importance of family and available networks in support relationships and emphasize the relative ineffectiveness of health factors as predictors of network size and composition.

Mullings L: Anthropological perspective of the Afro-American family, in The Black Family: Mental Health Perspectives. Edited by Fullilove MT. San Francisco, CA, Rosenberg Foundation, 1985, pp 11–21

The author discusses the African American family from an anthropological perspective. Various theoretical approaches to the African American family are reviewed as are the effects of their implementation as policy. The author critiques federal programs that emphasize a deficiency model of family function and exclude the effects of poverty and discrimination. Mullings then considers culture, class, and kinship; family structure; gender roles; and the contemporary African American family. He concludes by emphasizing the importance of reinterpreting and de-mythologizing the African American family in the context of the extensive theorizing concerning these families.

Taylor RJ: The extended family as a source of support to elderly blacks. Gerontologist 25:488–495, 1985

Taylor describes the complex extended family network of African American elderly and the determinants of the frequency of support, including income, education, degree of family interaction, and proximity of relatives.

Neighbors HW, Jackson JJ: The use of informal and formal help: four patterns of illness behavior in the black community. Am J Community Psychol 12:629–644, 1984

Most studies of African Americans who use professional help fail to describe this group's relationship to African Americans who are experiencing distress but are not requesting professional help, and generally ignore the salience of informal social support processes. A more comprehensive understanding of African American help-seeking behavior would come from an approach that describes both the users and nonusers of formal helping services, and that examines the benefits derived from kin-based networks. The article's analyses focused on four patterns of informal and formal help used based on the National Survey of Black Americans. The findings indicated that most people use either informal help only or a combination of informal and professional help. In addition, gender, age, income, and problem-type were significantly related to the differing patterns of illness behavior. The implications of these findings for help-seeking in the African American community are discussed.

Lewis JM, Looney JG: The Long Struggle: Well-Functioning Working Class Black Families. New York, Brunner/Mazel, 1983

This text describes the study of 18 working-class African American families in the inner city of West Dallas, Texas, by the Timberlawn Psychiatric Research Foundation. Combining statistical analysis with clinical profiles of these families, the authors effectively translate these data into human terms. Comparisons with the affluent (middle-class) white families studied in the book *No Single Thread* result in some interesting similarities as well as some significant differences in values and life-styles. The book described a longitudinal study of African American families with various economic resources resident in east

Dallas, Texas, a predominantly African American community. Examples of questions addressed by the study include the following: How does being African American and living in marginal economic circumstances affect what is possible in family life? How do economic and ethnic forces shape the structure and function of the family? How do some families manage to do very well despite a harsh environment?

Hines PM, Boyd-Franklin N: Black families, in Ethnicity and Family Therapy. Edited by McGoldrick M, Pearce JK, Giordano J. New York, Guilford, 1982, pp 84–107

Beginning with a cultural context and a discussion of kinship bonds and role flexibility, the authors continue with a discussion of several topical areas such as extended kinship networks and religion. Included are valuable case examples showing how a specific area was a key factor in family therapy. The impact of work and education on African American family members is presented. The chapter concludes with a discussion of specific ecological realities in the treatment of African American families and a consideration of the specific concerns and questions that African American family members bring to the treatment setting.

Jones BE, Gray BA, Jospitre J: Survey of psychotherapy with black men. Am J Psychiatry 139:1174–1177, 1982

The authors surveyed psychiatrists regarding psychotherapy with African American patients. Usable responses were received from 51 African American and 42 white psychiatrists; 99% of the African American psychiatrists and 48% of the white psychiatrists were currently treating African American patients. African American male patients were typically married, ages 31–40, had technical or semiprofessional occupations and some college education, sought treatment for depression or work-related problems, and remained in psychotherapy 13 weeks or more. Aggression/passivity was the most frequent unconscious conflict among the African American male patients; developing new coping mechanisms was the most difficult treatment state; and racism was often either a causative factor in the pathology or a symptom.

Seiden RH: Mellowing with age: factors influencing the non-white suicide rate. Int J Aging Hum Dev 13:265–284, 1981

Seiden presents data showing that although white elderly suicides increase with age, nonwhite elderly suicides decrease with age. Several hypotheses are discussed: less favorable life expectancies for nonwhites (survivor effects), the calming effects of the passing years (philosophical acceptance of hardships), greater respect for the elderly (status), maintenance of purposeful activities associated with age in nonwhites, and less "downward mobility" for nonwhites.

Stack C: All Our Kin. New York, Harper & Row, 1974

This brief book provides an in-depth look at the kinship network of African American families. The unique role of the African American elder is presented in a multigenerational context.

Jackson JJ: Sex and social class variations in black aged parent-child relationships. Aging and Human Development 2:96–107, 1971

Data were collected through personal interviews with 32 African American subjects in their seventies who were participating in the Duke University Longitudinal Geriatrics Project. These elders had a total of 83 living children (an average of 4.3 children per elder). Although most African American aged parents received some instrumental aid from their children, nonmanual parents (i.e., those providing moral support) were more likely than manual parents (i.e., those providing direct assistance) to receive such aid. Daughters were more likely than sons to provide such aid. Although most children of manual parents did not receive parental instrumental assistance, the opposite was true of children of nonmanual parents. (Daughters were more likely to receive aid from their nonmanual parents.) Nonmanual mothers received instrumental aid from their sons more often than any other group, followed by manual fathers receiving aid from their sons. In view of the controversy over matriarchy as the predominant African American family structure, the author indicated that this finding warranted further exploration. Most of these African American aged parents did not consider themselves or their children to be mutual sources of moral support. Usually, moral support and advice-giving in the sample tended to be reciprocated between a parent and child, and related positively as well, to the perceived degree of emotional closeness existing between a parent and child (as perceived by the parent). Further studies of African American elders and their children were encouraged.

Barriers to Care

Specific barriers to care in this cohort of elders are based on their prior experience of the segregation of health care facilities in their youth, the impact of lower socioeconomic status on knowledge of and access to psychiatric facilities, and attitudes toward the implications of acknowledging psychiatric symptoms or illness. Although the stigma associated with psychiatric illness is changing with increased public information, the African American elder is more likely to approach the health care system about psychiatric symptoms through a neighbor who is in the health care field or through the family physician.

The bias of the treating clinician for many years was a barrier to care and still may be of concern. If the African American patient was generally believed to be so "happy and carefree" that he or she could not become depressed, depression would not be diagnosed by a clinician sharing this belief. As racial prejudice affects diagnostic evaluation to a decreasing extent, the spectrum of psychiatric disorders is observed. Erroneous assumptions about the African American elder's ego strengths and psychological reserves by the therapist will hinder the development of a therapeutic alliance.

In working with African American elders, it is especially important to teach clinicians to explore the history of substance use, working conditions, and possible exposure to toxic chemicals more carefully. Psychiatric symptoms and disorders may result from trauma or exposure to work-related or illicit toxins. Even a past history of psychiatric problems recalled by the patient and his or her family may have been misdiagnosed. For example, many cases of affective disorder, organic mental disorders, substance abuse, and acute toxic psychosis have been mislabeled as schizophrenia.

Barriers to Care Bibliography

Baker FM: Ethnic minority elders: differential diagnosis, medication, treatment, and outcomes, in Minority Aging: Essential Curricula Content for Selected Health and Allied Health Professions (DHHS Publ No HRS-P-DV-90-4). Edited by Harper MS. Washington, DC, U.S. Government Printing Office, 1990, pp 549–577

The four groups of ethnic minority elders (African American, American Indian and Alaska Native, Asian American, and Hispanic American) are discussed in this chapter. The cultural values and historical context of an African American elder born in 1921 is reviewed. The elders' expectation of the health care system is acknowledged. The changing locus of mental health services from the community to the general hospital and community mental health center is presented. Specific issues of misdiagnosis and the range of psychiatric disorders present among African American elders are discussed.

Bradshaw MH: Training psychiatrists for working with blacks in basic residency training programs. Am J Psychiatry 135:1520–1524, 1978

The author provides residency training directors with recommendations for training psychiatric residents to work with African American and minority patients. The article stresses that therapists must engage in continuous introspection and self-analysis, must learn as much as possible about the culture of the patient, and must be keen to the external racist environment and the pressures to which the patient is exposed.

Jones A, Seagull A: Dimensions of the relationship between the black client and the white therapist. Am Psychol 32:850–855, 1977

The article provides a theoretical overview of the psychological issues involved in white therapists treating African American patients. One of the issues is the therapist's cognizance of his or her own feelings, countertransference, guilt, and the impact of his or her need as a therapist to be powerful. Another is the importance of the therapist's understanding of the different social system. The authors also explore the need for patient-therapist interpersonal similarity.

Schachter J, Butts H: Transference and counter-transference in interracial analysis. J Am Psychoanal Assoc 16:792–909, 1968

Some important racial occurrences in psychoanalytic treatment are that 1) racial differences may have little or no effect on the course of analysis; 2) racial differences may have a catalytic effect on the analytic process and lead to a more rapid unfolding of core problems; and 3) stereotypes of race and color occasionally induce both the analyst and the patient to delay the analytic process, either by obscuring reality or by overestimating its importance; 4) subculturally acceptable pathology or acting out may evoke overreactions in the analyst, whereas material fitting racial stereotypes may be ignored; and 5) counter-transference may coincide with stereotypes and delay in the analytic process.

Bevis WM: Psychological traits of the Southern Negro with observations as to some of his psychoses. Am J Psychiatry 1:76–78, 1921

The authors highlight the past ethnocentric bias affecting diagnosis and treatment, presenting "observations and deductions of phylogenetic traits of character, habit and behavior that affect psychoses in the Negro race." Statistics on psychotic disorders were gathered from southern state hospitals. Dementia praecox was the top in frequency, representing 698 of 2,732 admissions, and was thought to be due to the character makeup and superstition of the culture. One conclusion reads "most of the race are care-free with limited capacity to recall or profit by experiences of the past. Sadness and depression have little part in his psychological makeup. The number of cases of alcoholic psychoses [is] surprisingly low. Motion, rhythm, music and excitement make up a large part of the life of the race. . . . The manic phase [of manic-depressive psychosis] is the one nearly always seen. Nearly all psychoses of this race are dissociation, compensatory or repression types."

Jones BE, Gray BA, Jospitre J: Survey of psychotherapy with black men. Am
J Psychiatry 139:1174–1177, 1982

See p. 54 for annotation.

Clinical Treatment Issues

Because they lack contextual historical information about various African
American elderly groups, nonminority psychiatrists and treatment teams
often find it difficult to form a therapeutic alliance with an African American elder. The verbal and nonverbal behavior of the psychiatrist is often
evaluated by the elder for evidence of acceptance and interest, a test many
clinicians fail. The negative attitudes or mistaken stereotypes by clinicians
are a barrier that must be addressed by education. Nonminority clinicians
often overgeneralize from past experiences, invoking stereotypes about the
patient without obtaining detailed information about religion, mixed heritage, immigrant status, past employment status, upbringing, education,
and financial status. Some even attempt to be a "brother" or "sister" to the
patient and even attempt to use "black street talk" to establish rapport.
These countertransference problems can be minimized with appropriate
sensitization during training.

Past diagnoses must be questioned closely by a current psychiatrist,
particularly in light of the history of misdiagnosis of African Americans.
Even today, questions arise about racial differences in the range of doses
prescribed for psychoactive medications. Although studies in this area have
been completed for Asian elders, no published studies for African American elders are found to date. Special health risks for different treatments
may exist for African American elders. As in the case of Mr. J, presented at
the beginning of this chapter, impaired lithium clearance may exist for
patients with sickle-cell anemia or trait; a higher prevalence of slow acetylation in African Americans may affect the pharmacokinetics of psychoactive medications.

The need to work with immediate and extended families, friends,
fellow church members, and personal physicians of African American
elderly individuals appears to be more important than is the case among
nonminority patients. The illness and its course must be clarified to all

members of the African American elder's social network. Such an approach will facilitate the therapeutic alliance with the individual directly, as well as indirectly, by enlisting the support of the individual's network.

Clinical Treatment Issues Bibliography

Valle R: U.S. ethnic minority groups' access to long-term care, in International Long Term Care. Edited by Meyers T. New York, McGraw-Hill, 1988, pp 339–365

The author discusses access to long-term care services by ethnic minority populations, with an emphasis on principles for a proactive strategy to include culturally diverse populations in a redesigned long-term care system. Following a definition of *ethnic minority,* the author addresses the specific issues affecting access to long-term care by these elders. The chapter concludes with strategies for change that address structural considerations, an affirmative action stance, the provision of these services in ethnic communities, a focus on outreach and education to the community, and the importance of establishing a cross-cultural conceptual base.

Lawson WB, Yesavage JA, Werner PA: Race, violence, and psychopathology. J Clin Psychiatry 45:294–297, 1984

The article analyzes violent behavior among inpatients on an acute psychiatric unit for veterans. Compared with whites, African Americans were significantly less violent and less likely to commit multiple acts against others, although the actual numbers of violent episodes were not significantly different for the two races. No racial differences were noted in serum neuroleptic levels.

Shader RI: Cultural aspects of mental health care for black Americans: cultural aspects of psychiatric training, in Cross-Cultural Psychiatry. Edited by Gaw A. Boston, MA, John Wright, 1982, pp 187–197

This chapter adds another perspective to that of an earlier chapter that dealt with mental health issues for African American populations. The author addresses two key areas: recruitment of African American medical students and biological aspects of culture and ethnicity. Specific strategies for interesting students in medicine in general, and psychiatry in particular, are discussed. The author presents detailed tables containing the number of various minorities enrolled in medical school, the number of students repeating, the impact of the amount of time spent in a required clerkship, and choice of specialty. Early contact with undergraduate students is underscored as an important recruitment strategy. With respect to biological aspects of culture, the author notes that the proportion of individuals in the African American and white populations who are slow acetylators is about equal, around 55%. Slow acetylators will not metabolize a drug that requires acetylation and are at increased risk to develop systemic lupus erythematosis. Shader concludes by noting the developing literature that correlates early exposure to lead with lower adult cognitive function. Lead exposure will also increase the risk of lithium toxicity and irreversible nervous system disease.

Jackson JJ: The blacklands of gerontology. Aging and Human Development 2:156–171, 1971

This review article is a continuation of two previous critical reviews of selected literature pertinent to aging and aged African Americans. This article focuses largely on new data on health and longevity (including body age); psychology and race; and social patterns, policies, and resources. Because considerable attention has been given to investigations of the influence of race on aging and on differences among the African American aged, Jackson posits that two of the most critical research needs are in the areas of mental illness in the African American aged and trends in the use of nursing homes by the African American aged.

Conclusion

Although much has been written about African Americans, data about the elderly in this population are poor and still controversial. The mental health of elderly African Americans is affected by earlier onset of chronic disabilities and a culture of poverty for a large segment of the population. Mental health problems of this population have often been underestimated because of the relatively good mental health and constitutions of the elite group of "survivors" who do live beyond age 75.

Ethnocentric bias and stereotyping that have led to misdiagnosis have also clouded the findings of many early studies of African Americans. It is now well documented that depression and alcoholism have been underdiagnosed, and schizophrenia and cognitive impairment have been overdiagnosed, in this population. Today, problems of access to and acceptance of "traditional services" continue to plague the population. This is due partly to the long history of discrimination that has led to considerable suspicion about care and caregivers except in extreme mental health crises.

Reliable epidemiological data collection, controlled studies on racial differences in pharmacokinetics, concerted health education, better methods of establishing patient alliances, and ways to use the extended family network, will require in-depth exploration in both research and clinical practice.

Chapter 4

Issues in the Psychiatric Care of Hispanic American Elders

Richard G. Jimenez, M.D.
John M. de Figueiredo, M.D.

In his retirement, Mr. H, a 73-year-old Mexican attorney who retained many honorary positions within the business community, led an active and productive life. He had been an accomplished, respected lawyer and family patriarch. In the past year, however, family and professional colleagues noticed that Mr. H was becoming increasingly impaired. The burden of his worsening dependency led his family to urge that his condition be fully evaluated. An interview and examination revealed that Mr. H was addicted to and abusing a variety of anxiolytic and sedative-hypnotic medications. His apparent debilitation caused by the drug dependency was comparable to that found in cases of moderately advanced dementia. He was also found to suffer from clinically significant depression. After detoxification, rehabilitation, and stabilization with antidepressant medication, Mr. H's cognitive function and mood were significantly improved. During his hospitalization, Mr. H's wife had assumed many of his family responsibilities. When he returned home, he uncharacteristically resigned himself to a disempowered position and demonstrated no motivation to resume his former one. Despite efforts to address his issues in individual and family therapies, Mr. H "felt too old to make the effort."

Introduction

The Hispanic ethnic minority population, often referred to as *Latin Americans* or *Latinos*, actually consists of many cultural groups. Their cultural diversity in the United States arises partly from the different cultures of origin and partly from the different degrees of acculturation to, or assimilation of, Anglo-Saxon values. Information on the distribution of Hispanic Americans by the degree of acculturation, however, is largely unavailable. If Hispanics are arbitrarily defined as those individuals with Spanish surnames, the cultural diversity among them is enormous. Such a definition embraces immigrants from Spain, Mexico, Puerto Rico, Cuba, Central America, South America, and the Caribbean. Similarly, if Hispanics are defined as the Spanish-speaking people, the cultural diversity would be equally expansive. The different physical traits among Hispanics further complicate our efforts. Their ancestry may be of African, European (Italian, German, Spanish) or Native Indian descent. Thus, however we define this population, it remains broad and heterogeneous.

The United States has the sixth-largest Hispanic population in the world (Perez-Stable 1987). Hispanics are the second-largest minority group in the United States, accounting for 9% of the U.S. population in the 1990 census—22.4 million individuals (see Table 4–1 for a summary of Hispanic population characteristics from the 1990 Census of Population and Housing). Of this 9%, 60% are of Mexican origin, 12% of Puerto Rican origin, 5% of Cuban origin, and 23% of "other" Hispanic origin. Although generally a young group (38% under age 20 years, with a median age of 25 years), more than 1.1 million Hispanics are over age 65, constituting approximately 4.8% of the 31 million Americans 65 years or older in the United States. The Hispanic elderly are also the fastest-growing subgroup of the aged (Lopez-Aqueres et al. 1984). Between 1980 and 1990, the rate of increase in the U.S. Hispanic population increased at five times the rate of the total population (53% versus 9.8%).

Several criteria have been proposed and used to define *Hispanic* (e.g., those with Spanish surnames or those whose mother tongue is Spanish). No matter what the definition, Hispanic Americans constitute a broad, heterogeneous, and culturally diverse population. The cultural diversity arises partly from differences in the culture of origin and partially from variations in the degree of acculturation to or assimilation of Anglo-Saxon values. Information on the distribution of Hispanic Americans by the degree of acculturation, however, is largely unavailable.

In 1990, the mean household size for Hispanics was 3.53 members, slightly higher than that for all white persons (2.54). As of 1990, the median family income for all Hispanics was only $23,400, compared with $35,200 for the total population. The median family income per racial group was the following: Mexican origin, $23,400 (28.1% below the poverty line); Puerto Rican origin, $18,000 (40.6% below the poverty line); Cuban origin, $31,400 (16.9% below the poverty line); and Central and South American origin, $23,400 (25.4% below the poverty line). The number of Hispanics living below the poverty line (28% overall) was more than double that for the overall U.S. population (12.8%). Moreover, 26% of Hispanics have no medical insurance; 21% report having trouble with access to medical care.

Background Bibliography

Perez-Stable EI: Issues in Latino health care: medical staff conference. West J Med 146:213–218, 1987

A review of the demographic profile and historic roots of Latinos in the United States is provided. The problems in health care are assessed and

Table 4–1.   U.S. Hispanic population according to country of origin

Country or area of origin	Hispanic population			1990 median income (all ages; percentage below poverty level)
	Total	65 or older N	(%)	
Mexico	13,421,000	587,000	(4.4)	$23,240; 28.1
Puerto Rico	2,382,000	112,000	(4.7)	$18,008; 40.6
Cuba	1,055,000	156,000	(14.8)	$31,439; 16.9
Central or South America	2,951,000	89,000	(3.0)	$23,445; 25.4
Other	1,628,000	146,000	(9.0)	$27,382; 21.5

Source.   United States Bureau of the Census: *Statistical Abstract of the United States, 1992,* 12th Edition. Washington, DC, U.S. Department of Commerce, 1992.

the barriers to care are discussed. Special health risks of cardiovascular disease, tuberculosis, and depression are discussed with reference to proposals to develop effective health promotion programs.

Lopez-Aqueres W, Kemp B, Plopper M, et al: Health needs of the Hispanic elderly. J Am Geriatr Soc 32:191–198, 1984

This article presents results of a study concerning the health care needs of the Hispanic elderly population of Los Angeles County. Using the Comprehensive Assessment and Referral Evaluation (CARE) instrument, data on a sample of 704 subjects were employed to compute the scores for 22 Likert-type scales measuring the prevalence of numerous psychiatric, medical, and social problems. The data indicate that the older Hispanics were affected by cognitive impairment (18.8%), depression or demoralization (30.8%), heart disorders (12.8%), stroke effects (11.5%), arthritis (28.3%), hypertension (23.7%), financial hardship (28%), fear of crime (38.4%), ambulation problems (17.2%), and activity limitation (24.7%). They also needed assistance (19.3%) or used social services (22%). Further analysis revealed that the prevalence of many of these problems varied significantly according to the age, sex, language, and income of respondents. The indicators of health care needs used in the study differed substantially from the more traditional measures based on the individual's own perception of his or her health.

Bibliographical listings of special reports from the U.S. Bureau of the Census on persons of Spanish origin in the United States are listed in the General References section.

Diagnostic Differences

Some studies suggest that existing translations of standardized instruments, such as the Mini-Mental State Examination and the Minnesota Multiphasic Personality Inventory (MMPI), may not be valid for the Hispanic population. However, current studies are not definitive; more data are needed to validate or improve on both translated and untranslated forms of the various diagnostic instruments for the Hispanic population.

Studies on the presentation of psychiatric disorders are limited. Although Epidemiologic Catchment Area data (see Chapter 2) showed no higher incidence of major psychiatric disorders among Hispanics, other studies found higher psychotic-like symptoms; MMPI 2-7-8 configurations (schizotypal) profiles in low-acculturated Hispanics have been thought to be due to culturally normative beliefs or behavior patterns. Thematic Apperception Test studies in such individuals often show concreteness in perceptual cognitive patterns as well. Although there is little disagreement about the validity of diagnostic criteria for major psychiatric disorders such as schizophrenia, there are still disagreements over the existence of different, culturally based, diagnostic structures that are not captured by DSM-III-R–based mental health questionnaires (e.g., for dysthymia and possibly other diagnoses). Also, the distortion arising from the use of interpreters often leads to misdiagnosis of psychosis or dementia.

One published study suggests that biological markers for depression differ by race; few Hispanics show a response to the dexamethasone suppression test. Because many psychiatric symptoms have been linked to biological processes, the study implies that differences in symptomatology may be related to racial background. Further studies are needed.

Diagnostic Differences Bibliography

Wetle T, Schensul J, Torres M, et al: Alzheimer's disease symptom interpretation and help-seeking among Puerto Rican elderly. Geriatric Education Center Newsletter, The University of Connecticut Travelers Center on Aging 4(2):Winter, 1990

Data in this pilot study were derived from in-depth interviews conducted with 11 Puerto Rican elderly individuals (ages 66–82) and their caregivers. Because many symptoms were viewed as part of "normal aging" by both the elderly and their caregivers, few sought help for those disorders.

Hoppe SK, Leon RL, Realini JP: Depression and anxiety among Mexican Americans in a family health center. Soc Psychiatry Psychiatr Epidemiol 24:63–68, 1989

The sample consisted of adult patients (Mexican American, African American, and white) attending a county family health center in Texas. Presence of depression or anxiety was evaluated using the Diagnostic Interview Schedule (DIS). Although the mean age of patients was 49 years, many were 65 and above. Depression or anxiety was found in 14.3% of the women over age 65. The number of men in this age group in the clinic was too low to report. Significant differences were observed in the rates by sex, race, family integration, and physical status. Although age differences were not specifically analyzed by race, the study highlights the fact that there are differential rates of mental disorders due to sociocultural determinants that need more detailed examination.

Liang J, Tran VT, Krause N, et al: Generational differences in the structure of the CES-D in Mexican Americans. J Gerontol 44 (social sciences suppl):S110–S120, 1989

The usefulness of the Center for Epidemiologic Studies—Depression Scale (CES-D) scale in assessing depressive symptoms in groups other than white and African Americans is still not well established. The authors interviewed 375 respondents in each of three generations of Mexican Americans in San Antonio, Texas, using the CES-D, and looked at potential measurement error and structural variations in responses across generations and among levels of acculturation. In a statistical sense, convincing differences were noted in the measurement of error variances for all generations, although the greatest disparity was between the first and second generations. The findings do not negate the use of the CES-D for screening purposes, but the "second-order" depressive factors of psychological distress and positive well-being could have a different meaning for those populations.

Espino DV, Neufeld RR, Mulvihill M, et al: Hispanic and non-Hispanic elderly on admission to the nursing home: a pilot study. Gerontologist 28:821–824, 1988

The records of all Puerto Rican/Hispanic patients ($N = 25$) residing in, or discharged within the last 12 months from, a nursing home were reviewed and compared with a control group ($N = 50$) admitted during the same period. The Puerto Rican/Hispanic group was younger and had a greater number of disabilities. Their families were not able to maintain an impaired member at home, which contradicts the common view that Puerto Rican/Hispanic families refuse to use nursing homes.

Mahard RE: The CES-D as a measure of depressive mood in the elderly Puerto Rican population. J Gerontol 43:24–25, 1988

This study assessed the validity of the Center for Epidemiologic Studies-Depression Scale (CES-D) using a sample of 60 elderly Puerto Ricans in New York City, half of whom were diagnosed as clinically depressed. The scale was found to have high internal consistency and reliability, to discriminate strongly between patients and nonpatients, and to relate in the expected fashion to theoretically relevant variables. There is some evidence that scores are influenced by socially desirable responding; these effects should be considered when examining the correlates of the CES-D in this population. Scale scores do not differ by interviewer. Overall, the CES-D appears to be a useful measure for studying within-group variability in depressive mood among older Puerto Ricans.

Mendes deLeon C, Markides KS: Depressive symptoms among Mexican Americans: a three-generational study. American Journal of Epidemiology 127:150–160, 1988

The distribution of depressive symptoms and rates of high depressive symptomatology are examined using Center for Epidemiologic Studies-Depression Scale data from a three-generation study of 1,074 Mexican Americans that was conducted in San Antonio, Texas, in 1981 and 1982. Associations between sociodemographic variables and depressive symptoms were similar to those in earlier studies, although this sample experienced comparatively low levels of depressive symptoms, particularly among males. Interactions may exist between generations and other relevant variables typically found to be related to distribution of depressive symptoms in the general population.

Bernstein IH, Teng G, Grannemann BD: Invariance in the MMPI's components structure. J Pers Assess 51:522–531, 1987

The authors examined whether the representation of the Minnesota Multiphasic Personality Inventory (MMPI) clinical scales using a three-component structure (i.e., profile evaluation, test-taking attitudes, optimism-pessimism) generalizes across sex and race. The MMPI scores of Hispanics, whites, African Americans and Native Americans were analyzed. The salient weight model and the principal component structure remained invariant across race, sex, and context for test-takers (i.e., job applicants vs. inmates). Several alternative definitions of profile elevation were found to provide equally satisfactory representation of the relations among the MMPI scales.

Bird H, Canino G, Stipec MR, et al: Use of the Mini-Mental State Examination in a probability sample of Hispanic population. J Nerv Ment Dis 175:731–737, 1987

The Diagnostic Interview Schedule (DIS) was applied to 1,532 subjects ages 18–64. The prevalence of severe cognitive impairment was found to be significantly higher than that reported in similar studies in U.S. communities.

Burnam M, Hough R, Escobar J, et al: Six-month prevalence of specific psychiatric disorders among Mexican Americans and non-Hispanic whites in Los Angeles. Arch Gen Psychiatry 44:687–694, 1987

In this study the prevalence of phobia and obsessive-compulsive disorder was lower in Los Angeles than in two other sites. Non-Hispanic whites had higher rates of drug abuse or dependence than did Mexican Americans. Mexican Americans displayed higher rates of severe cognitive impairment, a finding that likely reflects ethnic and educational bias in the measurement of cognitive impairment. Another ethnic difference was found for one specific age and sex group; Mexican American women, 40 years of age and older, had strikingly high rates of phobia.

Karno M, Hough R, Burnham M, et al: Lifetime prevalence of specific psychiatric disorders among Mexican Americans and non-Hispanic whites in Los Angeles. Arch Gen Psychiatry 44:695–701, 1987

The lifetime prevalence of DSM-III–defined psychiatric disorders among 1,243 Mexican American and 1,309 non-Hispanic white residents of Los Angeles is reported from the Los Angeles sites of the Epidemiologic Catchment Area research study. Non-Hispanic whites reported far more drug abuse or dependence and more major depressive episodes than Mexican Americans. Alcohol abuse or dependence was highly prevalent among Mexican Americans and non-Hispanic white men of any age. Mexican American women infrequently abused or became dependent on drugs or alcohol at any age. Dysthymia, panic disorder, and phobia were somewhat more prevalent among Mexican American women over 40 years of age than among non-Hispanic white women in the same age group and Mexican American women under 40.

Kemp BJ, Staples F, Lopez-Aqueres W: Epidemiology of depression and dysphoria in an elderly Hispanic population: prevalence and correlates. J Am Geriatr Soc 35:920–926, 1987

Depression in the elderly in minority groups, including Hispanics, has not been well studied. Little is known of depression: its rate, its correlates, and how well it is treated. This study is part of a series examining health status of older Hispanics using the Comprehensive Assessment and Referral Evaluation (CARE). A sample of 700 elderly Hispanics living in Los Angeles County were selected using an area-probability sampling method. The CARE items were regrouped to reflect DSM-III criteria for depression and dysphoria. Over 26% of the sample was found to suffer major depression or dysphoria. These affective disorders were strongly correlated with physical health status. In the absence of physical health complications, the rate was 5.5%. A number of socioeconomic, health behavior, and family variables were related to affective state. Treatment for affective disorder appeared to be very poor for this population.

Escobar JI, Burnam A, Karno M, et al: Use of the Mini-Mental State Examination (MMSE) in a community population of mixed ethnicity: cultural and linguistic artifacts. J Nerv Ment Dis 174:607–614, 1986

The Mini-Mental State Examination was used in an epidemiologic survey of a community of mixed ethnicity (Hispanic, non-Hispanic white) as part of the Los Angeles Epidemiologic Catchment Area study. Results of the study showed that age, educational level, ethnicity, and language of the interview influenced the number of MMSE errors. Items on which the effects of ethnicity and language were most pronounced are identified, and suggestions on ways to minimize such sociocultural artifacts are provided to improve the epidemiologic significance of the instrument, particularly as it concerns cross-cultural research.

Neff JR: Alcohol consumption and psychological distress among U.S. Anglos, Hispanics and blacks. Alcohol Alcohol 21:111–119, 1986

The study analyzed data from the Health and Nutrition Examination Survey Augmentation Component conducted by the National Center for Health Statistics in 1978 to assess differences in alcohol use and psychological distress among 5,546 whites, 872 African Americans, 182 less-acculturated Hispanics, and 58 more-acculturated Hispanics. Subjects were ages 25–75. Results indicate that quantitative differences in alcohol consumption were more notable than frequency differences. Hispanics reported significantly higher consumption quantities than did whites or African Americans. White and African Americans who drank were more depressed than were individuals of the same ethnic origin who did not drink. Interestingly, an opposite but insignificant pattern emerged among Hispanics. Use of higher quantities of alcohol was generally associated with greater depressive symptomatology and lower well-being; higher frequency of alcohol use was generally associated with lower depressive symptoms and higher well-being.

Swanda R, Kahn M: Differential perception of life crisis events by sex, diagnosis, and ethnicity in rural mental health clients. Journal of Rural Community Psychology 7:63–68, 1986

A sample of 146 rural mental health patients ranging from ages 16 to 66 years were studied. Significantly different life-stress event statements were elicited from Hispanic Americans than from European Americans.

Escobar JI: Are results on the dexamethasone suppression test affected by ethnic background? Am J Psychiatry 142:268, 1985

A sample of 142 subjects (ages 20–76 years) received a 1-mg dexamethasone suppression test (DST) as part of a routine evaluation at a Veterans Administration outpatient clinic. Sixty-five subjects were minority members, including 42 Hispanic Americans, 32 African Americans, and 4 Asian Americans. Data show that 33 subjects were DST nonsuppressors; 18 of 46 subjects with DSM-III-R primary major depressive disorder were nonsuppressors. By race, 32% of white, 19% of African American, and 14% of Hispanic subjects were nonsuppressors. Among those diagnosed with major depressive disorder, 58% of whites were nonsuppressors. In contrast, only 25% of African Americans and none of the Hispanics with major depressive disorder were found to be nonsuppressors. These findings suggest that ethnic background may affect DST results.

Randolph ET, Escobar JI, Paz DH, et al: Ethnicity and reporting of schizophrenic symptoms. J Nerv Ment Dis 173:332–340, 1985

Using a structured interview, the National Institute of Mental Health Diagnostic Interview Schedule (DIS) and a battery of rating instruments (Brief Psychiatric Rating Scale, Clinical Global Impression Scale, Global Impression Scale, and the Symptom Checklist-90 [SCL-90]), the authors evaluated 40 white and 41 Hispanic clinically diagnosed schizophrenic subjects (ages 20–42 years). The study examined the consistency in symptom reporting across different instruments administered in different formats, and evaluated the effect of ethnic background on that consistency. A subgroup of subjects (23% of total) denied lifetime schizophrenic symptoms in the lay interviewer-administered structured interview (DIS-negative subjects). The proportion of DIS-negative subjects was similar across the two ethnic groups.

However, Hispanic and white DIS-negative subject responses were significantly different on the SCL-90. A subgroup of white subjects denied symptoms on the DIS, but volunteered symptoms on the self-rating instrument. Responses of Hispanic subjects were consistent regardless of format.

Fuller CG, Malony HH: A comparison of English and Spanish (Nunez) translations of the MMPI. J Pers Assess 48:130–131, 1984

The authors investigated the validity of the Nunez-published—and most widely used—Spanish translation of the Minnesota Multiphasic Personality Inventory (MMPI). Both the Nunez translation and the English MMPI were administered to a volunteer sample of 18 bilingual Hispanic young women (ages 14–18). A split-plot factorial analysis of variance with one between-subject factor (form of test) was used to analyze the K-corrected T-scores from each scale. On scales F, K, HS, PA, and SC, the Spanish means were significantly higher than the English means. Order of administration had no significant effect; no significant interaction effect was detected. These findings demonstrate that the Nunez translation cannot be used interchangeably with the English MMPI.

Bozlee S: A cross-cultural MMPI comparison of alcoholics. Psychol Rep 50:639–646, 1982

The study compared Minnesota Multiphasic Personality Inventory (MMPI) profiles of 11 white, 11 Hispanic American, and 11 American Indian men with alcoholism, ages 25–76. One-way nonrepeated measure analyses of variance on validity and clinical scales as well as the MacAndrew Alcoholism Scale showed significance only for scale 2 scores, which were elevated, but within the normal range for the Hispanic American group. Resultant profiles conform to previous MMPI prototypes for alcoholism, supporting the use of the MMPI for the populations studied. Results do not support the development of separate MMPI norms for psychiatric subjects from these minority groups.

Price CS, Cuellar I: Effects of language and related variables on the expression of psychopathology in Mexican American psychiatric patients. Hispanic Journal of Behavioral Sciences 3:145–160, 1981

Thirty-two patients (ages 24–28) diagnosed with schizophrenia participated in an investigation of the effect of interview language on the expression of psychopathology and its relationship to verbal fluency, acculturation, and self-disclosure. Subjects were interviewed twice, once in Spanish and once in English; videotapes were rated independently by bilingual mental health professionals using the Brief Psychiatric Rating Scale to determine the extent of psychopathology expressed by the subjects during each interview. Subjects expressed more symptomatology indicative of psychopathology during the Spanish interview. Verbal fluency, acculturation, and self-disclosure were a significant combined predictor of the difference between expressed psychopathology in the English and Spanish interviews. Verbal fluency and acculturation were also unique predictors of this difference.

Hates-Bautista DE: Identifying "Hispanic" populations: the influence of research methodology upon public policy. Am J Public Health 70:353–356, 1980

This excellent editorial examining various criteria used to define the Hispanic population clarifies population definition for future research and public policy activities.

Marcos LR: Effects of interpreters on the evaluation of psychopathology in non-English-speaking patients. Am J Psychiatry 136:171–174, 1979

Non-English-speaking patients in need of psychiatric services are usually evaluated using an interpreter. Discussions with psychiatrists and lay hospital interpreters experienced with these interviews, coupled with content analysis of eight audiotaped interpreter-mediated psychiatric interviews, suggested that clinically relevant interpreter-related distortions could lead to misevaluation of a patient's mental status. The author notes that pre- and postinterview meetings of clinicians and interpreters have been found useful in minimizing these distortions.

Health and Mortality Issues

Among the Hispanic elderly, mental health and well-being are strongly related to physical health status. Unfortunately, morbidity and mortality data are limited, in part because national reporting systems have not listed Hispanics as an ethnic group separate from other whites. A recently completed Hispanic National Health Examination and Nutrition Survey provides the most comprehensive health morbidity data available. The health of Hispanics is closer to that of other whites than to African Americans with whom they share socioeconomic conditions. Life expectancy and infant mortality rates among Hispanics are nearly equivalent to those of whites; cardiovascular disease mortality and cancer incidence rates are lower among Hispanics than among whites. Hispanics, however, face higher rates of diabetes, obesity, alcohol-related illness, and mortality from homicide than found in the general population. The homicide rate among Hispanics is lower than among African Americans.

Nineteen percent of Hispanics, in contrast to 13% of whites, report no routine source of medical care. Many more—26%—have no medical insurance, nearly triple the 9% of whites without insurance. The percentage of Hispanics with no physician contacts during the year preceding an interview in 1979–1980 was higher for Mexican Americans (33.1%) than for other Hispanics (23.3%) and for whites (23.3%). In 1982, 21% of the Hispanics polled reported difficulty in gaining access to medical care. Some could not find services, were refused care, could not afford care, or simply did not seek care. The same survey reported that 13% of whites had similar difficulties with service access.

Life expectancy at birth for Hispanics in the Southwest is nearly the same as for other whites in the same region. A California study found life expectancy of men with Spanish surnames to be 68.3 years, compared with 68.7 years for other whites. Women with Spanish surnames had a life expectancy of 75.2 years, compared with 76.0 years for other whites.

Data indicate that the prevalence of diabetes among Mexican Americans is nearly twice that found among whites (11.6% of men; 9.8% of women), more than 95% being non-insulin dependent. Diabetes among Mexican Americans of low socioeconomic status appears to be more than twice as common as it is among those of high socioeconomic status. The incidence of cancer among Hispanics appears to be lower than that of other whites. Obesity is a problem in 25.9% of men and 44.9% of women, 2–4 times higher than the white general population.

A 1979–1981 study of Hispanic areas of Los Angeles County showed that age-adjusted mortality rates from major cardiovascular disease were lower for Hispanic men than for white or African American men (441.9 deaths per 100,000 compared with 536.2 and 558.2, respectively). Hispanic women also had lower age-adjusted cardiovascular disease-related mortality rates than white or African American women (316.7 per 100,000 compared with 333.5 and 384.4, respectively). Nonetheless, two studies found cardiovascular disease to be the leading cause of death among Mexican Americans in the Southwest. The Hispanic suicide rate in the five Southwestern states in 1976–1980 was less than half the rate among other whites. In a 1981 California survey, a higher percentage of Hispanic men (24%) reported frequent heavy drinking than did other white (21%) or African American (21%) men. A higher percentage of Hispanic women (33%) reported abstinence than did other white (18%) or black (32%) women. The prevalence of obesity in those of low socioeconomic status is higher among Mexican American men (25.9%) and women (44.9%) than in non-Hispanic white men (15.6%) and women (29.0%). Several studies have found the prevalence of high blood pressure to be similar among Hispanic Americans and other whites.

Health and Mortality Issues Bibliography

Trevino FM (ed): Hispanic Health and Nutrition Examination Survey, 1982–1984: findings on health status and health care needs. Am J Public Health 80:(entire volume), 1990

The volume summarizes findings from the Hispanic Health and Nutrition Examination Survey (HHANES) related to the effects of acculturation and generational differences on access to care and preventive health services, health risk behaviors, use of Curanderos, alcohol consumption patterns, cigarette smoking patterns, marijuana and cocaine use, and dental care. A selective bibliography of HHANES publications citing 60 additional health references is listed. None of the references deals directly with the mental health of the elderly Hispanics in the survey.

Furukawa C, Harris MB: Some correlates of obesity in the elderly: hereditary and environmental factors. Journal of Obesity and Weight Regulation 5:55–76, 1986

The authors examined variables associated with obesity in a survey of 208 adults (ages 42–94)of whom 78% were white and 14% were Hispanic. Subjects completed an anonymous questionnaire including demographic data, information about health-related characteristics, knowledge measures, personal attitudes toward obesity, and experience with physicians (including the physicians' attitudes toward obesity). Results showed that obesity, as measured by body mass index, was negatively correlated with age, education, and frequency of exercise. It was correlated positively with number of overweight relatives and with snacking. Body mass was not significantly related to marital status, sex, caloric intake, or health problems (with the exception of arthritis). Hispanics were more obese than whites and were more often advised to diet. Subjects were reasonably knowledgeable about obesity, related health problems, and caloric values of foods. However, such knowledge was unrelated to body mass.

Markides KS, Coreil J: The health of Hispanics in the Southwest U.S.: an epidemiological paradox. Public Health Rep 101:253–265, 1986

Recent reports in the literature on the health status of Southwestern Hispanics, most of whom are Mexican Americans, are reviewed critically. The review is organized into the following sections: infant mortality, mortality at other ages, cardiovascular diseases, cancer, diabetes, other diseases, and interview data on physical and mental health. Despite methodological limitations of much of the research, it can be concluded with some certainty that the health status of Hispanics in the Southwest is much more similar to the health status of other whites than it is to that of African Americans, although socioeconomically, the status of Hispanics is closer to that of African Americans. This observation is supported by mortality data, life expectancy, mortality rates from cardiovascular disease, mortality rates from major types of cancer, and measures of functional health. On other health indicators, such as diabetes and infectious and parasitic diseases, Hispanics appear to be clearly disadvantaged when compared with other whites. Factors explaining the relative advantages or disadvantages of Hispanics include cultural practices, family supports, selective migration, diet, and genetic heritage. The recently completed Hispanic Health and Nutrition Examination Survey will go a long way to provide answers to many questions regarding the health of Hispanics in the Southwest and elsewhere.

Smith JC, Mercy JA, Rosenberg ML: Suicide and homicide among Hispanics in the Southwest. Public Health Rep 101:265–270, 1986

A study of suicide and homicide among Hispanics of Mexican origin focused on five Southwestern states—Arizona, California, Colorado, New Mexico, and Texas—where more than 60% of all Hispanics in the United States reside. Of these, 85% are Mexican Americans. Although specific age breakdowns are not provided, the suicide rate per hundred thousand for Hispanics (9.0) was less than the national rate for whites (13.2) and half that of the whites residing in the same area (19.2). For homicide, the overall rate per hundred thousand for Hispanics (20.5) was more than two-and-a-half times that of whites (7.9).

Kosten T, Rounsaville B, Kleber H: Ethnic and gender differences among opiate addicts. Int J Addict 20:1143–1162, 1985

The authors studied a population of 522 opiate-addicted subjects (ages 18–65). Opiate addicted Puerto Ricans in the study population were found to have the highest rate of unemployment; the least education; the greatest amount of poly-drug abuse and violent crimes; and the highest rates of schizophrenia, anxiety disorders, and neurotic or depressive symptoms.

Lopez-Aqueres W, Kemp B, Plopper M, et al: Health needs of the Hispanic elderly. J Am Geriatr Soc 32:191–198, 1984

A sample of 700 Hispanic elderly (ages 60+) were studied. Thirteen percent of the study population was found to be affected by cognitive impairment. The authors found the prevalence of psychiatric, medical and social problems to vary by age, sex, language, and income. (This reference was also discussed earlier on p. 66.)

Special Areas of Concern

The major mental health concerns of the Hispanic elderly result from the residual effects of the pre–civil rights era and the consequences of historical discrimination and segregation. These antecedents of the health status of Hispanic elderly individuals has only recently been addressed through the evolution of public policy. Health, self-esteem, hope, knowledge, and trust in the care system have all been affected by the life experiences of the Hispanic elder.

Special Areas of Concern Bibliography

Kutza EA: A policy analyst's response. Gerontologist 26:147–149, 1986

The author comments on articles by Dressel, Hess, Watson, and Torres-Gil that examine whether civil rights legislation will improve the life chances of elderly black and Hispanic men and women in the future. Kutza concludes that such an analysis may be premature and misleading, because the life chances of future elderly are more likely to be affected by policies other than affirmative action.

Torres-Gil F: An examination of factors affecting future cohorts of elderly Hispanics. Gerontologist 26:140–146, 1986

The author reviews trends in the Hispanic population, including future socioeconomic position based on evaluation of educational, occupational, income, and pension data. Civil rights legislation appears to have had limited effect in reducing multiple jeopardies for today's elderly Hispanics; it may have even less effect in reducing discrimination for future cohorts.

Maldonado D: The Hispanic elderly: a socio-historical framework for public policy. J Appl Gerontol 4:18–27, 1985

Maldonado discusses the Hispanic contribution to the formation of the United States as a multiethnic entity, and examines issues and concerns of older Hispanics arising from their experiences of foreign birth and immigration, minority status in the pre–civil rights era, World War II, the social reform of the 1960s, and postreform trends. He reports that as the result of conquest and discrimination, Hispanics have been subjected to minority status with limited use of national resources. Older Hispanics, products of the pre–civil rights era, enter old age with the social and physical consequences of historical discrimination and segregation. Thus, they are among the most vulnerable of the older population.

Family and Support Issues

The family support systems of Hispanic groups differ by ethnic subpopulation and may not decrease in importance for each generation removed from the point of immigration as in many other ethnic groups. The extended family has a strong impact on service use by Hispanic elderly, although the diversity of family and extended-family supports among Hispanic groups have made generalizations to all Hispanics difficult.

Family and Support Issues Bibliography

Greene VL, Monahan DJ: Comparative utilization of community-based long-term care services by Hispanic and Anglo elderly in a case management system. J Gerontol 39:730–735, 1984

The authors compare use of formal and informal supports by 21 Hispanic and 87 white elderly enrollees in a comprehensive case management system. On average, Hispanics used significantly fewer agency services than did whites, despite a tendency to exhibit higher levels of impairment. However, Hispanics used significantly higher levels of informal support, possibly a mediating factor in their lower use of agency services.

Weeks JR, Cuellar JB: Isolation of older persons: the influence of immigration and length of residence. Res Aging 5:369–388, 1983

Current theories suggest that migration tends to exacerbate the isolation experienced by older people; such isolation, however, should be mitigated by length of residence. Propositions derived from these theories were tested using data collected in San Diego from 1,139 individuals (ages 55 and over) representing 10 different ethnic groups. The findings suggest that elderly recent immigrants are more isolated than other elders. However, immigration seems to exert less overall influence on isolation than does the fact of ethnicity itself.

Mindel CH: Extended familism among urban Mexican Americans, Anglos, and blacks. Hispanic Journal of Behavioral Sciences 2:21–34, 1980

In semistructured interviews, measures of familism (i.e., presence of and relationships with nuclear and extended family members in the community) were evaluated for 143 white, 160 African American, and 152 Mexican American adults in families with at least one child in parochial or public elementary school. Mexican Americans had the highest levels of extended familism and whites the least. Analysis of the effects of migration indicated that whites moved away from the kin network, whereas Mexican Americans moved toward or within the network. Patterns among African Americans were in between those of the other two populations.

Barriers to Care

Most studies in this area reveal the significance of barriers between patient and provider created by differences in language, cultural relevance, needs, and ethnicity. Other practical difficulties encountered by ethnic elderly individuals in need of psychiatric care include a lack of information about providers, distance from services, and cost. The overreliance on purported respect for elders in an ethnic subculture may contribute to policy errors and inadequate services for Hispanic elders.

Barriers to Care Bibliography

Greene MG, Adelman R, Charon R, et al: Ageism in the medical encounter: an exploratory study of the doctor-elderly patient relationship. Language Communication 6(1–2):113–124, 1986

Physician language and behavior were studied to test the hypothesis that doctors relate differently to young and old patients. Five physicians from medical outpatient programs of a large urban hospital were audiotaped while interviewing four elderly and four young patients who were age and sex matched. The Geriatric Interaction Analysis Tool was used to evaluate physician approaches. More medical and fewer psychological issues were discussed in interviews with elderly patients, surprising in view of the authors' expectation that loneliness would cause elderly patients to see a doctor for nonmedical reasons. Better questioning, information, and support were provided by the physicians to the younger patients. Overall, subjects were significantly more egalitarian, patient, engaged, and respectful when treating younger patients. Ageism appears to exacerbate the passivity of the patient role.

Garcia JL: A needs assessment of elderly Hispanics in an inner city senior citizen complex: implications for practice. J Appl Gerontol 4:72–85, 1985

To provide better services to the Hispanic elderly population, the author sought to determine the needs of this population in the Tampa Bay, Florida, area by obtaining information on their perceived needs, awareness of community services, and perceived extent to which needs were being met. A bilingual questionnaire was developed and administered in Spanish to 45 elderly residents (ages 62–85) of an inner-city retirement facility in a predominantly Hispanic neighborhood. Results show service gaps in health care, finance, and support for specific tasks of daily living. The majority of subjects were unaware of most community resources; pride, communication difficulties, and fear of being poorly received limited their use of known services. Problem areas are discussed and recommendations are made on the assessment of, and service delivery to, ethnic groups.

Sokolovsky J: Ethnicity, culture and aging: do differences really make a difference? J Appl Gerontol 4:6–17, 1985

The author examines the effect of cultural differences on the elderly, drawing on cross-cultural generalizations about aging that are relevant to understanding the ethnic aged in the United States. The author focuses on the extent to which overidealization of ethnic subcultures has resulted in policies that rely on informal caregiving within the ethnic family for the care of the elderly. This issue is examined as it relates to a variety of ethnic groups: Italian, Irish, Polish, African American, Hispanic, and Asian American.

Marin BV, Marin G, Padilla AM, et al: Utilization of traditional and nontraditional sources of health care among Hispanics. Hispanic Journal of Behavioral Sciences 5:65–80, 1983

One hundred low-income Hispanics (ages 16–72) were interviewed about patterns of health care use and perceptions of health service use by members of their community. Responses showed substantially low rates of use of preventive services, although most subjects knew when care should be sought. Few subjects used folk providers. Financial difficulty was the most significant reason given by subjects for having never visited a private physician or dentist. When asked to rate why people do not receive appropriate care, subjects specified economic difficulties and insurance as the most important reasons, followed by such system barriers as lack of child care, time conflicts, and language barriers.

Dolgin D, Grossner R, Cruz-Martinez S, et al: Discriminant analysis of behavioral symptomatology in hospitalized Hispanic and Anglo patients. Hispanic Journal of Behavioral Sciences 4:329–337, 1982

The authors studied a population of 100 individuals (ages 18–59) residing in a state-run psychiatric facility and concluded that socioeconomic conditions alone did not explain the prevalence of mental illness within the Hispanic inpatient population. Communication difficulties and resistance to the hospital milieu were hallmark issues for the Hispanic inpatients.

Vandenbos GR, Stapp J, Kilburg RR: Health service providers in psychology: results of the 1978 APA Human Resources Survey. Am Psychol 36:1403–1426, 1981

The study presents data on health service provider psychologists (HSPs) extracted from a larger 1979 study of a stratified random sample of 6,551 American Psychological Association members. Of all the HSPs, 83.8% held a doctoral degree, 71.1% were male, and 84.3% of doctoral HSPs were licensed. Minority doctoral-level HSPs included African Americans (1.1%), Hispanics (0.9%), Asian Americans (1.0%), and Native Americans (0.2%). Examination of practice location revealed that 64% of all sampled were primarily employed in organized settings; 24% were engaged in private practice. Information on population of service area and type of community is presented. The average doctoral HSP spent 21.1 hours per week in direct clinical care. In addition, 11.2% of the clinical services delivered were to children (ages 11 and under), 12.4% to adolescents (ages 12–17), and 2.7% to the elderly (ages 65 and over), with the balance of services provided to adults ages 18–64. The most frequent type of service provided was individual psychotherapy, followed by assessment and diagnosis, and consultation.

Gaviria M, Stern G: Problems in designing and implementing culturally relevant mental health services for Latinos in the U.S. Soc Sci Med 14:65–71, 1980

Hispanics, the fastest growing minority in the United States, have consistently underused mental health services. Three constituencies active in planning mental health services for Hispanic populations are government funding agencies, social scientists, and Hispanic activists. Each has approached the issue of cultural relevance in mental health service delivery from a different perspective. A case study illustrates the difficulty of implementing and defining ultimately relevant services in a Mexican American community mental health center. Directions for future research to develop and evaluate culture-specific treatment modalities are suggested.

Szapocznik J, Lasagna J, Perry P, et al: Outreach in the delivery of mental health services to Hispanic elders. Hispanic Journal of Behavioral Sciences 1:21–40,1979

This study investigates two ways to increase use of mental health services by Hispanic elders. Outreach through the mass media was found to be the more effective of the two.

Clinical Treatment Issues

Articles and books in this area are sparse. Clinical work with Hispanic elderly individuals has many potential pitfalls for therapists who are not culturally sensitive or trained. Some of the considerations for both group and individual work include the therapist's possible authority patterns of counseling and the patient's immediate and extended family network, attitudes toward caretakers, transference themes, and communication and cognitive manifestations of being multilingual. Often, a clinician's view of the Hispanic elderly population as poorly motivated or difficult to treat can be overcome through cultural sensitivity training.

Clinical Treatment Issues Bibliography

Comas-Dias L: Puerto Rican alcoholic women: treatment considerations. Alcoholism Treatment Quarterly 3:47–57, 1986

The author describes the culturally relevant clinical treatment of five Puerto Rican alcoholic women (ages 19–54) in a group setting. An educational component consisting of didactic sessions on alcoholism, stages of alcoholism, alcohol and nutrition, and physical consequences of alcohol specific to women was added to the treatment plan. The group setting was complemented by the inclusion of significant others in the treatment. Given the difficulties in attracting Puerto Rican alcoholic women into treatment, the author urges education and prevention of alcoholism among Puerto Rican women.

Minrath M: Breaking the race barrier: the white therapist in interracial psychotherapy. J Psychosoc Nurs Ment Health Serv 23:19–24, 1985

The author suggests that racial and ethnic stereotyping is a defensive maneuver used by both patient and therapist to cope with the anxiety aroused by the interracial nature of the relationship. The reflective process of analyzing his or her feelings and reactions to the ethnic minority patient can help the white therapist cope with conflicts presented in interracial psychotherapy. The therapist's exploration of the patient's cultural background through inquiry about customs, lifestyle, language, and use of idioms express the therapist's desire to learn about and understand the sociocultural world of the patient. Case histories of two African American men (ages 16 and 28), a 35-year-old African American woman, and a 24-year-old Puerto Rican woman are presented to illustrate the importance of accepting a patient's individuality in the development of the interracial therapeutic relationship.

Franklin GS: Group psychotherapy for elderly female Hispanic outpatients. Hosp Community Psychiatry 33:385–387, 1982

The author describes the establishment of a successful group psychotherapy program for eight depressed and anxious elderly Hispanic females (ages 60–72). The program was designed to facilitate symptomatic relief, establish more gratifying relationships with family and friends, and provide a more positive experience within the clinical setting.

Gonzalez DVA, Usher M: Group therapy with aged Latino women: a pilot project and study. Clinical Gerontologist 1:51–58, 1982

The authors describe the formation of a therapy group for aged Hispanic women and discuss the external and internal threats to the group's purpose. Hispanic cultural factors and their relevance for group therapy are identified: authority patterns in counseling, the disintegration of the extended family, attitudes toward caretakers, and implications for transference. Suggestions are made for improvement.

Tylim I: Group psychotherapy with Hispanic patients: the psychodynamics of idealization. Int J Group Psychother 32:339–350, 1982

The author discusses transference and idealization among Hispanic patients based on 3 years of therapist observation. Hispanic patients in group therapy seek emotional refueling from the omnipotent lost parental object. Groups conducted in Spanish seem to unveil an idealized transference that condenses the pull of regression with the high respect the Hispanic holds for the authoritarian figure. An early rapport in these groups generally permits regression to early stages of object relations. It is common for Hispanics to join a group soon after returning from a visit to their homeland or shortly after arrival in the United States. The proximity of the homeland affects the patient's way of handling termination and separation issues. The bonds formed by the almost-instant rapport of these groups lead to strong transferential links and to primitive defense mechanisms. Narcissistic transference is important because it helps fill the gap left by the loss of the old omnipotent object. Idealizing transference occurs when the patient begins to view the therapist as a parent or perfect person.

Szapocznik J, Santiseban D, Herris O, et al: Treatment of depression among Cuban-American elders: some validational evidence for a life enhancement counseling approach. J Consult Clin Psychol 49:752–754, 1981

Szapocznik reports outcome research on a counseling approach developed to provide an age-appropriate and culturally sensitive treatment model to alleviate depression among Cuban American elders. Sixty-six subjects (average 67.2) were administered the Older American Resource Scale Multidimensional Functional Assessment Questionnaire and the Subjective Distress Macroscale of the Psychiatric Status Schedule. Treatment outcome analysis indicated significant improvement in functioning along all dimensions evaluated. Additional analyses were performed to identify patient and treatment variables that were differentially predictive of treatment success.

Marcos LR, Alpert M: Strategies and risks in psychotherapy with bilingual patients: the phenomena of language independence. Am J Psychiatry 133:1275–1278, 1976

The presence of two separate languages, each with its own lexical, syntactic, semantic, and ideational components, can complicate psychotherapy undertaken with proficient bilingual patients. If only one language is used in therapy, some aspects of the patient's emotional experience may be unavailable to treatment; if both languages are used, the patient may use language switching as a form of resistance to affectively charged material. The authors suggest that monolingual therapists should assess the degree of independent areas of use for each language in bilinguals to minimize its impact on therapy. They conclude that study of bilingual patients may provide important insights into the nature of the therapeutic process.

Conclusion

Low-acculturated Hispanic elderly patients present linguistic and financial barriers to care, different belief systems, and life-styles that can lead to physical illness. On the basis of such culturally based presenting factors, non-Hispanic clinicians may misdiagnose these patients. Despite the huge differences among Hispanic groups in the United States, most studies lump Hispanic groups for analysis. It is a policy error to base decisions about needs of the Hispanic elderly on current data, which are sparse and inconsistent. Prejudice and discrimination from the dominant white population have led to considerable socioeconomic strain for many Hispanic families, leading to the inability to care for the elder.

Chapter 5

Issues in the Psychiatric Care of American Indian and Alaska Native Elders

James W. Thompson, M.D., M.P.H.

A 63-year-old Cherokee woman was brought to the Indian Health Service (IHS) clinic by her son and daughter-in-law. They informed the IHS physician that over the last 6 months, the patient, who lived alone in the Ozark Mountains of Oklahoma, had become more and more suspicious of people outside her family and at times had "talked crazy." During the last 2 weeks, she had refused to leave her house; the son feared that she had stopped eating. After much urging, she agreed to visit a medicine woman in the community, who performed a ceremony and also suggested the patient be taken to the IHS clinic.

Introduction

Manson and Pambrun (1979) note a general omission in the gerontological literature: "the elderly in question are usually white, seldom black, and

The author greatly appreciates the assistance of the National Center for American Indian and Alaska Native Mental Health Research, Denver, CO, and its director, Spero Manson, Ph.D.

In this review, *Indian* refers to the indigenous peoples of mainland North America, including Canadian Indians and Alaska Natives. Hawaiian natives are not included only because no literature was available.

never Indian." With few exceptions, little has changed in the past decade. Literature on the elderly American Indian is very sparse indeed; studies of specific psychiatric issues arising in this population are nearly nonexistent. What literature does exist is often difficult to locate, because few studies appear in major journals. We simply do not know about the overall psychiatric status of the Indian elder—what diagnostic and treatment differences from the general population may exist or what level of access to care is available to this population. Although model programs of care have been set in place, most have not been evaluated or described in the literature.

Most researchers believe that the psychiatric disorders most common among the Indian elderly are depression, somatization, and organic mental disorders (Cross P, Manson S, Westermeyer J, personal communications, 1989). However, a nursing home study (Mick 1983) suggests that the prevalence of organic mental disorders among Indian elders in that setting may be lower than among the dominant cultural and ethnic groups in the United States.

Certain areas appear nearly entirely overlooked in the literature. First, an informal survey of clinicians, researchers, and administrators engaged in work with Indian elders suggests that alcoholism studies have been seriously neglected. The prevalence of alcoholism among the Indian elderly has not been established, although limited literature suggests the prevalence to be lower than is found among younger age groups. Second, elder abuse has not been studied. The Indian population has a long history of honor for elders. However, as that tradition wanes, the threat of elder abuse grows. The implications for psychiatric disorders have not been investigated.

Recognizing the narrow and shallow research base from which to draw, we have, nonetheless, attempted to extract information from all extant literature in the field. A few works included in this annotated bibliography do not discuss Indian elders per se, but do illustrate a particular syndrome or problem. Others are even more tangential to the field. We have chosen to err in favor of being overinclusive. Clearly, the field is wide open for research and clinical reports.

A major problem in the literature is the diversity of the Indian population. Several hundred tribal or cultural groups are found in North America. Although some commonalities among the groups exist, many differences are also present. This is made more complex by the impact of the majority culture, which also varies within tribal groups and between individuals within tribal groups. Researchers in this field face a choice between validity and generalizability. If we study a single tribal group, we cannot make statements about the overall population; if we combine statistics from many groups, we sacrifice validity. The literature contains examples of each. Articles based on specific tribes generally are impressionistic, with few statistical inferences possible. National data provide little insight into psychiatric issues confronting individual elders from a particular area or tribe. Our ability to improve the current base of literature on the Indian elder will depend on our ability to overcome this basic problem.

Diagnostic Differences

Few studies have examined the efficacy of existing diagnostic tools and strategies in the care of older Indian individuals. What little work has been undertaken has related mainly to depression. Baron et al. (1990) focused on the Indian elderly in a study that evaluated whether the National Institute of Mental Health Center for Epidemiologic Studies–Depression Scale (CES-D) is a useful diagnostic screening tool for Indian elders with chronic disease. Goldstine and Gutman (1972) undertook a Thematic Apperception Test study of Navajo aging. Kunitz and Levy (1988) report that "mind loss" is thought by one tribe to be the final stage of all disease.

Perhaps the best examples of the types of research necessary for an understanding of psychopathology in Indians is the work of Shore et al. (1987) and Manson et al. (1985). In this study, Indian subjects were given a standard diagnostic instrument. Diagnostic differences in depression between Indian populations and non-Indians were found to be minimal. However, the overall paucity of literature underscores the need for much more data examining diagnostic issues among Indians in general and Indian elders in particular.

Diagnostic Differences Bibliography

Baron AE, Manson SM, Ackerson LM, et al: Depressive symptomatology in older American Indians with chronic disease: some psychometric considerations, in Screening for Depression in Primary Care. Edited by Attkisson C, Zich J. New York, Routledge, Chapman & Hall, 1990, pp 217–231

The Center for Epidemiologic Studies–Depression Scale (CES-D) was tested as a screening tool in three tribal groups. The subjects were Indian elders with chronic diseases ($N = 314$). Internal consistency of the instrument was good. Sensitivity was 100%, but specificity was 73% compared with DSM-III and 71% compared with the Research Diagnostic Criteria. The study uncovered few false negatives, supporting the use of CES-D in preventive intervention or other screening strategies. The authors note, however, that use of this tool as a diagnostic instrument is not advised pending further study.

Manson SM, Moseley R, Brenneman D: Physical illness, depression, and older American Indians: a preventive intervention trial, in Special Populations: Preventive Intervention Concerns: A New Beginning. Edited By Owan T, Silverman M. Washington, DC, U.S. Government Printing Office (in press)

This article was originally presented at the 1984 conference, "Medical Anthropology: Implications for Stress Prevention Among Culturally Different Populations," Portland, Oregon. It describes a study that targeted interventions for high-risk Indian elders, ages 50 and older, in the northwest United States. *High risk* was defined as the presence of a deteriorating physical health condition. The intervention was a psychoeducational course on coping with depression. The authors describe the pretest-posttest design and the outcome measures of depressive symptomatology and individual coping skills. However, the article does not report study results.

May PA: Mental health and alcohol abuse indicators in the Albuquerque area of the Indian Health Service: an exploratory chart review. American Indian and Alaska Native Mental Health Research 2:33–46, 1988

This article, based on a 10-year chart review in one Indian Health Service area, is perhaps the only longitudinal account of inpatient and outpatient visits for psychiatric disorders by Indian people. Both general medical records and mental health program records were reviewed. Analysis of general medical charts disclosed that alcohol and drug overdose headed the list of disorders, followed by conversion reaction, adjustment disorders in adolescents, anxiety, depression, adolescent antisocial behavior, and "victim of sexual assault." The category of hypertension is included, somewhat inexplicably. Review of the mental health program charts yielded all of the foregoing diagnoses as well as family and marital problems, schizophrenia, neuroses, and personality disorder.

Shore JH, Manson SM, Bloom JD, et al: A pilot study of depression among American Indian patients with Research Diagnostic Criteria. American Indian and Alaska Native Mental Health Research 1:4–15, 1987

This outstanding and unusual article describes the administration of a standard diagnostic instrument to Indian subjects in three different tribal cultures. The results indicated that depressive diagnoses differed little among the three tribes and followed a pattern similar to that in the majority culture. The diagnostic subgroups identified in the study included 1) uncomplicated pattern of depression, 2) secondary depression with a history of alcoholism, and 3) complicated depression superimposed on an underlying chronic depression or personality disorder. The authors note that choice of treatment options may vary not only by diagnostic subtype but also by culture. This study is worth repeating across many tribal cultures, age groups, and diagnostic categories.

Manson SM, Shore JH, Bloom JD: The depressive experience in American Indian communities: a challenge for psychiatric theory and diagnosis, in Culture and Depression. Edited by Kleinman A, Good B. Berkeley, CA, University of California Press, 1985, pp 331–368

The authors present both a well-documented review of depression in Indian people and a study attempting to determine how a particular tribe, Hopi, conceptualizes depression. Based on their findings, the authors construct a culturally appropriate instrument to be used in the diagnosis of depression in Hopi culture. At the time of the article's publication, the instrument (American Indian Depression Scale) was being administered to a sample of Hopis. The authors discuss some preliminary findings. Although it does not focus on the elderly, this study exemplifies the type of research required to enhance understanding of psychopathology in Indians.

Kunitz SJ: Disease Change and the Role of Medicine: The Navajo Experience. Berkeley CA, University of California Press, 1983

Kunitz makes many interesting points, though neither specific to the Indian elderly nor generalizable to other tribes. He suggests, however, that the elderly represent a growing proportion of hospitalized patients, and discourses briefly on the question of home care versus institutionalization. One of the most interesting points made regarding diagnosis is the belief among some Navajos that "mind loss" (e.g., as in faints, dissociative reactions, seizures) is the end stage of all disease.

Author's note. This might imply that for the Navajo, mental disorder is not seen as something to be "treated." Because it is the end stage of all illnesses, perhaps it is seen as occurring after all hope of cure is lost. This has not been verified, however.

Manson SM, Shore JH: Psychiatric epidemiological research among American Indians and Alaska Natives: methodological issues. White Cloud Journal 2:48–56, 1981

This article reviews three community-based epidemiologic studies of Indians and discusses many of the methodological questions that arise in conducting such studies. It does not focus on the elderly, but serves as a model of how future epidemiologic studies of Indian elders might be conducted.

Shore JH, Manson SM: Cross-cultural studies of depression among American Indians and Alaska Natives. White Cloud Journal 2:5–12, 1981

A review of the literature on depression in Indians, this article also includes a short description of culture-bound syndromes. Although not focused on the elderly, the material presented has relevance for future work specific to the aging Indian population.

Westermeyer J, Walker D, Benton E: A review of some methods for investigating substance abuse among American Indians and Alaska Natives. White Cloud Journal 2:13–21, 1981

This article reviews the literature on substance abuse research among Indians. As with Shore and Manson (1981), the work does not focus on the elderly but is relevant as a model for future investigations.

Rhoades ER, Marchall M, Attneave CL, et al: Impact of mental disorders upon elderly American Indians as reflected in visits to ambulatory care facilities. J Am Geriatr Soc 28:33–39, 1980

Ambulatory Patient Care forms and the mental health and social services data base from the Portland and Albuquerque Indian Health Service areas are presented and analyzed. Although the data pose methodological problems, the authors carefully interpret the data in light of them. However, notwithstanding their own assessment that the data underrepresent the prevalence of psychiatric problems among Indian elders, they state that because of low service use by the elderly, the "lack of interest in mental health in aging may be justified."

Association of American Indian Physicians: Report on Physical and Mental Health of Elderly Indians. Final report of a contract with the Indian Health Service. Rockville MD, Indian Health Service, U.S. Public Health Service Health, Education, and Welfare, 1978

Prepared for a 1978 conference on the Health of Elderly American Indians (in Billings, Montana), the report indicates that the medical problems of elderly Indians are not necessarily unique to their culture. For example, visits for the treatment of schizophrenia did not appear to differ from those of the majority culture. Manic-depressive psychosis, however, may be lower in the Indian elderly population than in the majority culture. Alcoholism was found to diminish with age. (Because these statements are based on treated cases, they should not be confused with rates of illness derived from community samples.) The report concludes that culture-specific mental health screening and testing instruments must be developed, that risk factor research must be conducted, that data must be gathered to facilitate service planning and multicultural research, and that preventive programs must be developed and established.

Goldstine T, Gutman D: A TAT study of Navajo aging. Psychiatry 35:373–384, 1972

This Thematic Apperception Test (TAT) study compares Navajo men ages 35–54 to Navajo men ages 55–95. The findings are similar to those found in other cultures and ethnic populations. The authors attempt to determine the relative roles of acculturation and age in differences found between the older and younger group.

Indian Health Service: Chart Book Series. Rockville, MD, Program Statistics Branch, Indian Health Service, Department of Health and Human Services (published annually)

This series of publications includes data on Indian health by age, but not by psychiatric diagnosis. Suicide and homicide statistics are included. The rate of suicide for elderly Indians (over age 55) is lower than that for all races combined, for both men and women; it is roughly comparable to rates for non-Indian minority groups. Homicide is higher among Indian men and women than among whites, but lower than among other minority groups. Automobile-accident and other accident rates are much higher for elderly Indians (both sexes) than for all races combined. The overall death rate for elderly Indians is lower than that found in all non-Indian minority populations combined.

Health and Mortality Issues

This section of the annotated bibliography includes many references for conference reports that have made important recommendations for the care of Indian elders. A number of areas in need of attention are set forth repeatedly: long-term care (see Manson 1989 for an excellent overview); culturally relevant programs; coordinated mental health, general health, and social services programs; and the need for better integration of the elderly into their communities.

Health and Mortality Issues Bibliography

Manson SM: Provider assumptions about long-term care in American Indian communities. (unpublished manuscript)

The author surveyed 208 Indian Health Service (IHS) providers and discovered that they subscribed to the myths that long-term care and nursing home care are synonymous, that long-term care is rendered predominantly by formal health care professionals, and that the care is only rehabilitative and protective in nature. Manson underscores the need for more extensive geriatrics training of IHS personnel. Mental health services are mentioned only in the context of the benefits of and need for better integration of mental health with general health and social services.

Manson SM, Heegard W: Urban Indian health care: the Portland program and patient population. Med Anthropol (in press)

This article reports on a study of 62 patients randomly chosen from the population at the Portland Area Urban Health Clinic. Approximately one-third of the subjects were elderly. The clinic was found to be the primary source of all health care for the majority of the study population. The study surveyed basic health needs, care-seeking behavior, and service use. Gaps in service and barriers to care delivery are discussed.

Manson SM: Long-term care in American Indian communities: issues for planning and research. Gerontologist 29:38–44, 1989

In this article, oriented toward general health issues, the author discusses planning and research needs in the delivery of long-term care to the American Indian population. Manson believes that the Indian Health Service (IHS) has resisted the development of elderly-specific services, particularly those related to long-term care. He notes that

American Indian communities are between 10 and 15 years behind the majority culture in the construction of nursing homes. Nationally, only 10 reservation nursing homes—a total of 435 beds—are functioning, generally providing only one level of care. Manson notes that IHS physicians "seldom provide even minimal care within these nursing homes" and then suggests the need for more intensive research examining institutional care and community- and home-based services for Indian communities.

Joos SK, Ewart S: A health survey of Klamath Indian elders 30 years after the loss of tribal status. Public Health Rep 103:166–173, 1988

This article reviews the health of the elders (ages 40 and over) of a tribe that, in 1954, lost its federal recognition and with it all federally supported health, education, and welfare services. In 1985, the authors undertook a health status and health care needs assessment using a shortened version of the Older Americans Resources and Services instrument ($N = 202$). Of the Klamaths surveyed, 20% reported diabetes; more than 30% reported arthritis, rheumatism, hypertension, or gall bladder removal. The data were compared with those gathered using the same instrument in national surveys of Indian and non-Indian elders. Although the Klamaths surveyed were younger than the comparison groups, their health status was no better than that of other Indians and was worse than that of the non-Indian population. Moreover, Klamath adults had lower levels of health insurance coverage and greater perceptions of unmet health care needs than were found in the comparison groups. Mental disorders were not included as a survey topic.

Kunitz SJ, Levy JE: A prospective study of isolation and mortality in a cohort of elderly Navajo Indians. Journal of Cross-Cultural Gerontology 3:71–85, 1988

Largely concerned with predictors of mortality, the study tested 271 elderly Indian subjects over a 3-year period with a modified Diagnostic Interview Schedule to learn more about depressive symptoms in the population. Unfortunately, the article presents no research results.

Montgomery RJ, Borgatta EF, Kamo Y, et al: A profile of Alaska's seniors: income, children, and health. Res Aging 10:534–549, 1988

This demographic profile also discusses issues of life satisfaction. Although not specific to mental health and illness issues, it does contain some discussion relevant to these matters. The article represents one of the very few about elderly Alaska Natives that is found in medical, psychological, and social welfare literature.

Taylor TL: Health problems and use of services at two urban American Indian clinics. Public Health Rep 103:88–95, 1988

This article compares health problems of, and primary health care service use by, a sample of American Indians with national and regional data that had been compiled on Indian and majority populations by the Indian Health Service, the U.S. Bureau of the Census, the Office of Technology Assessment, and the National Center for Health Statistics. A survey of medical records was conducted at urban Indian health clinics in Oklahoma City and Wichita ($n = 500$ records per clinic). These data suggested that the clinics' clientele had annual incomes well below the average income found in both the general population and in the overall Indian population in these cities. Use of primary health care services was lower than that by the general population but comparable to that by American Indians living in rural Oklahoma and Kansas. Medical records review yielded high levels of diabetes mellitus and hypertension among middle-age groups, and high levels of contraceptive and prenatal care by young women. Only 81 subjects were ages 65 and over. Surprisingly, no medical records listed a psychiatric disorder as the reason for the clinic visit. It is possible that a bias toward identifying a "physical" reason for a visit is reflected in this finding.

United States Congress, Office of Technology Assessment: Indian Health Care (Publ No OTA-H-290). Washington, DC, U.S. Government Printing Office, 1986

This is perhaps the most exhaustive analysis of the Indian health care system. It contains a great deal of data, much of it age-adjusted.

Shah CP, Farkas CS: The health of Indians in Canadian cities: a challenge to the health care system. Can Med Assoc J 133:859–863, 1985

A general review of the literature about urban Canadian Indian health, this article does not focus specifically on the elderly or on mental disorders. It includes discussion of health problems and health service use (including some discussion of substance abuse, suicide, depression, anxiety, and family crises). The authors make reference to a number of U.S. studies, identify existing health care programs, and discuss sociocultural barriers to care. The report recommends further research into epidemiology and access to care of urban Canadian Indians, including the efficacy of collaborations with local Indian organizations.

Timpson JB: Indian mental health: challenges in the delivery of care in northwestern Ontario. Can J Psychiatry 29:234–241, 1984

Although not specific to the elderly, this article presents an interesting picture of the use of psychiatric and nonpsychiatric consultants, and indigenous counselors in the management of mental and emotional problems of Canadian Indians. Because the majority of cases were being managed by nonpsychiatrists, the identified presenting problems in the population were predominantly mild (e.g., 29% were identified as marital difficulties). Of particular interest, a small percentage of presenting problems were described as "problems associated with aging." The article also provides a detailed portrait of a service program.

Mick C: A Profile of American Indian Nursing Homes. Tucson, AZ, Working Paper and Reprint Series, Long-Term Care Gerontology Center, University of Arizona, 1983

Eight Indian nursing homes are characterized and compared with non-Indian nursing homes. Within the Indian nursing homes, the number of male patients is equal to or greater than the number of female patients, in sharp contrast to non-Indian nursing homes. Other comparisons yield interesting findings: the prevalence of an alcoholism history and sequelae of alcoholism (particularly for men) was substantially higher, and the rates of cognitive impairment significantly lower, than that among non-Indian nursing home patients.

National Indian Council on Aging: Indian Elders: A Tribute—Final Report of the Fourth National Indian Conference on Aging. Washington, DC, National Indian Council on Aging, 1982

Specific recommendations are made for improving health and mental health services for the Indian elder. Recommendations for mental health are comparable to those made in previous National Indian Conferences on Aging (1976, 1978, and 1980).

Young TK: Self-perceived and clinically assessed health status of Indians in northwestern Ontario: analysis of a health survey. Can J Public Health 73:272–277, 1982

The author reports on a community health interview survey and clinical examination undertaken in a 20% stratified random sample (stratified by community) in 25 Indian reservations in northwestern Ontario accessible only by air. Of 1,053 respondents, 45 were ages 65 or older. Seventy-three percent of the elders reported illness during the 2 weeks prior to the survey and examination. Most symptoms reported became more common with increased age. The single most common psychiatric problem mentioned in the interviews was alcohol use; 20% of those over age 15 reported alcohol use; only 4.6% of the elderly said they drank.

National Indian Council on Aging: American Indian Elderly: A National Profile. Washington, DC, National Indian Council on Aging, 1981

This volume provides general but useful information on the Indian elderly.

White House Conference on Aging: The American Indian and Alaska Native Elderly. Technical Report. Washington, DC, U.S. Government Printing Office, 1981

Among other findings, the report indicates that 4,600 elderly Indians resided in non-Indian nursing homes, most of which were located far from the patients' home communities. Few elderly Indians were found in any single non-Indian nursing home. Not surprisingly, visits from relatives were less frequent than among the overall resident population. Activity patterns and dietary habits of the elderly Indian residents were possibly quite different from those of other patients. (Reported in Manson 1989; see p. 99.)

National Indian Council on Aging: May the Circle Be Unbroken: A New Decade—Final Report on the Third National Indian Conference on Aging. Washington, DC, National Indian Council on Aging, 1980

Specific recommendations are made in this report for improving health and mental health services for the American Indian elder. Recommendations for mental health are similar to those recommendations made in previous National Indian Conferences on Aging (1976, 1978).

Manson SM, Pambrun AM: Social and psychological status of the American Indian elderly: past research, current advocacy, and future inquiry. White Cloud Journal 1:18–25, 1979

This general article, emphasizing mental health issues, traces the history of the National Indian Council on Aging and summarizes the mental health issues that arose during two national Indian conferences—Indians and Aging (Arizona State University, 1975) and First National Indian Conference on Aging (Phoenix, Arizona, 1976). A short literature review includes some otherwise unavailable citations. The authors conclude that the literature is heavily psychoanalytic, descriptive, and based on nonrepresentative information. The article includes discussion of the authors' own study, a questionnaire investigation in which the subjects were self-selected and the return rate was 20%. The emphasis of the study was on satisfaction with community response to the American Indian elderly, not on psychiatric issues.

Focus on native health. Can Nurse 74(9):8–9, 1978

An introduction to a journal issue devoted in part to Indian health, the article is a general statement on the health condition of Canadian Indians. It notes several studies that have shown that Canadian Indians have high rates of mental health problems, specific diseases, injuries, infant deaths, and hospital admissions. The article suggests that cultural differences have created barriers to the use of health care facilities, and identifies low socioeconomic status, cultural differences, and discrimination as primary impediments in cities to adequate health care and good health. The elderly are not discussed per se in this article.

Obomsawin R: A statement on Indian health (editorial). Can Nurse 74(9):7, 1978

This one-page statement, written by the health coordinator of the National Indian Brotherhood of Canada, explicates the conflict between Indian and white cultures, and the illnesses that have resulted among the Indian population. Although not wholly germane to issues of the Indian elderly, it is a stirring statement of the Indian ways of · health.

National Indian Council on Aging: The Continuum of Life: Health Concerns of the Indian Elderly—Final Report of the Second National Indian Conference on Aging. Washington, DC, National Indian Council on Aging, 1978

Specific recommendations are made for improving health and mental health services for the Indian elder. Recommendations include development of and access to senior citizen centers; provision of local, on-site, or live-in care; maintenance of the Indian cultural heritage through education, including multigenerational experiences in which the elders may teach younger generations; use of nursing homes (preferably on or near reservations) only as a treatment site of last resort; provision of whole-person treatment specific to the elderly; and development of community-based programs to curb alcohol and drug abuse and to protect community members from dangers posed by those using such substances.

American Indian Nurses Association: Alternatives for Planning and Continuum of Care for Elderly American Indians. Final Report to Fulfill a Contract With the Indian Health Service. Rockville, MD, Indian Health Service, U.S. Public Health Service, Department of Health, Education, and Welfare, 1978

This report was prepared for a 1978 conference on the Health of Elderly American Indians (Billings, Montana). The report recommends culturally relevant homemaker and home health, day care, and residential services. The need for tribe-initiated community programs for the elderly is discussed, as is the need to train professionals and others working with this diverse population to recognize and meet its special needs.

National Indian Council on Aging: The Indian Elder, a Forgotten American. Final Report of the First National Indian Conference on Aging. Washington, DC, National Tribal Chairman's Association, 1976

The report makes specific recommendations for improving health and mental health services for the Indian elder. These include efforts to foster activities important to physical, spiritual, and cultural well-being; to ensure continued community involvement by elders; to promote provision of social services by indigenous personnel; to promote training of Indian staff to provide home-based services as an alternative to nursing home care; and to use indigenous staff to work in alcohol abuse programs targeted to Indian populations using traditional healing methods.

French J, Schwartz DR: Terminal care at home in two cultures. Am J Nurs 73:502–505, 1973

The authors describe two approaches to care for the terminally ill: one found in the Navajo culture and one in the Italian culture. The use of a psychiatric consultant to the terminally ill Navajo is mentioned. The article emphasizes the importance of understanding the patient's cultural base and provides a description of the interface of Navajo culture with Western medical practice.

White House Conference on Aging: Report on the Special Concerns Session on the Elderly Indian. Washington, DC, U.S. Government Printing Office, 1971

Although cited in other literature, this report appears to be unavailable from standard reference sources and the U.S. Government Printing Office.

Surgeon General of the United States: Health Services for American Indians, Surgeon General's Report to Congress (PHS Publ No 531). Washington, DC, U.S. Public Health Service, Department of Health, Education, and Welfare, 1957

This report was completed immediately after the Public Health Service became responsible for Indian health care. The National Institute of Mental Health prepared the section on mental health issues. The elderly are not mentioned, per se, but some of the report's recommendations are relevant to this population—specifically, the need for epidemiologic data, culturally relevant mental health training for Indian Health Service personnel, increased consultation and treatment for the mentally ill and mentally retarded, mental health programs that are integrated with general health and social services programs, and mental health programs that are approved by tribal leaders.

Presentation of Psychiatric Disorders

The literature contains limited information concerning the presentation of psychiatric disorders in Indian cultures. Among the existing works, few pertain to the elderly. This section of the bibliography presents a number of articles that inform about syndromes thought by some to be culture bound. However, Manson and others have suggested that the concept of culture-bound syndromes may be a reasonable research construct, but is of limited help in the clinical setting. A practitioner may view such a syndrome as outside the bounds of medicine and may fail to evaluate psycho-pathology that is well within the realm of the practitioner's expertise (see Manson, unpublished manuscript, see below). The reader is also directed to the section on diagnostic differences, which contains references that question whether presenting symptomatology is different for American Indians and non-Indian populations.

Presentation of Psychiatric Disorders Bibliography

Manson SM: Physicians and American Indian healers: issues and con-straints in collaborative health care. (unpublished manuscript)

> In this outstanding article that emphasizes mental health issues, Man-son reviews native healers and healing, and their relationship to West-ern caregivers and medicine. He reviews how native healers, once considered by Western thinkers to be mentally ill themselves, are now viewed as skillful practitioners able to collaborate with Western medi-cal personnel. He provides accounts of both successful and unsuccess-ful collaborations, raising such issues as disparate definitions of illness and the concept of culture-bound syndromes as possible explanations for failed collaborations. Although elders are not considered per se, this work presents many insights into treatment needs of the Indian elder, since traditional healing is of significant importance to this population.

Shore JH, Manson SM: Cross-cultural studies of depression among Amer-ican Indians and Alaska Natives. White Cloud Journal 2:5–12, 1981

> See Diagnostic Differences section for annotation (p. 96).

Lewis TH: A syndrome of depression and mutism in the Oglala Sioux. Am J Psychiatry 132:753–755, 1975

> The article presents a case report on *wacinko*, a form of reactive depres-sion in a 63-year-old woman. The article emphasizes the need for the Western psychiatrist to work with native herbalists in the treatment of this disorder.

Jelik WG, Todd N: Witchdoctors succeed where doctors fail: psychotherapy among the Coast Salish Indians. Canadian Psychiatric Association Journal 19:351–356, 1974

The article describes how the perception of the native healer has changed from one of "crazy witch doctor" to one of "auxiliary psychotherapist."

Special Areas of Concern

The paucity of literature on the American Indian elder is epitomized by the near absence of material concerning psychiatric research on this population. The information that exists tends to be anecdotal and predominantly sociological. Many issues are in need of concerted psychiatric research activity:

- ✦ The relationship between psychiatric disorder and elderly Indians' belief systems about mental and physical illness, health, and the life cycle
- ✦ Long-term care (community- and institution-based)
- ✦ Elder abuse and the role of the elder in the community
- ✦ Substance abuse by the elder; substance abuse by family members and the impact on the elder
- ✦ Somatization as a symptom of psychiatric illness
- ✦ Use of traditional healing and Western medical techniques

Family and Support Issues

National conferences centering on Indian elderly issues (see Health and Mortality section for references, p. 99) have yielded many recommendations to address questions about family and support. Few studies have examined these issues; even fewer have a psychiatric focus.

Family and Support Issues Bibliography

Shomaker DJ: Transfer of children and the importance of grandmothers among the Navajo Indians. Journal of Cross-Cultural Gerontology 4:1–18, 1989

This article discusses the role of informal "grandmothers" in caring for Indian children whose parents cannot. Both the stresses placed on such older women and the mechanisms of these intergenerational relationships are discussed.

John R: Service needs and support networks of elderly Native Americans: family, friends, and social service agencies, in Social Bonds in Later Life: Aging and Interdependence. Edited by Peterson WA, Quadagno J. Beverly Hills, CA, Sage, 1985, pp 229–247

This chapter reports data from the 1980 National Council on Aging survey and addresses, in part, mental health and health care seeking issues.

Manson SM, Callaway DG: Problematic Life Situations: Cross-cultural Variation in Support Mobilization Among the Elderly. Final report on Grant Number 0090-AR-0037. Administration on Aging, 1984

The authors indicate that older urban Indians ($n = 76$) and older reservation Indians ($n = 155$) perceive physical illness and limitations stemming from related disabilities as the most difficult of life situations. Although social networks appear to be both willing and able to help, the study suggests that many elders perceive such "helpers" to lack the resources needed to provide effective assistance (from Manson 1989; see Health and Mortality Issues section).

Strong C: Stress and caring for elderly relatives: interpretations in coping strategies in an American Indian and white sample. Gerontologist 24:251–256, 1984

The study presents the findings of structured interviews with a small sample of Indians and non-Indians and notes population differences in the definition of caretaker responsibility, the locus of control, and the perception of caretaker stress.

Porter D: Mental health treatment and prevention: focus on elders, in Colloquium on American Indian Families: Developmental Strategies and Community Health. Edited by Mitchell W, Red Horse J. Phoenix, Arizona State University School of Social Work, 1982, pp 12–27

The author presents recommendations regarding the availability of safe and comfortable housing, the delivery of health support services (e.g., household chore assistance, visiting health and nutrition), community programs on aging, special mental and general health programs for the elderly, community support systems, legal services, and long-term care. Special mention is made of the problem of nursing home care provided away from the reservation.

American Indian Nurses Association: The Environment of Elderly Native Americans. Final report of a contract with the Indian Health Service. Rockville, MD, Indian Health Service, U.S. Public Health Service, Department of Health, Education, and Welfare, 1978

This report prepared for a 1978 conference on the Health of Elderly American Indians (Billings, Montana) makes a number of recommendations in such areas as living facilities, sanitation, transportation, nutrition, legal assistance, protective services, culture, information and referral services, and recreation. The authors state that such services should be coordinated through a core agency.

Barriers to Care

No references specific to barriers to care were found in the literature. However, a few articles cited in other sections of this chapter describe impediments to both access and delivery of needed services.

Manson SM, Heegard W: Urban Indian health care: the Portland program and patient population. Med Anthropol (in press)

Shah CP, Farkas CS: The health of Indians in Canadian cities: a challenge to the health care system. Can Med Assoc J 133:859–863, 1985

Focus on Native Health. Can Nurse 74(9):8–9, 1978

Clinical Treatment Issues

The literature on diagnosis is sparse, and on clinical treatment it is almost nonexistent. Although there is every reason to believe that treatments of mental disorders that are efficacious for the non-Indian elderly will also be found to be effective for the Indian elderly, this proposition has been seldom studied. Equally, the hypothesis that traditional Western treatments will not work for Indian populations has not been evaluated. In addition to the single reference that follows, treatment issues have been mentioned in several articles in the Diagnostic Differences section of this chapter.

Clinical Treatment Issues Bibliography

Manson SM, Callaway DG: Health and aging among American Indians: issues and challenges for the biobehavioral sciences, in Behavioral Health Issues Among American Indian and Alaska Natives (American Indian and Alaska Native Mental Health Res Monogr No 1). Edited by Manson SM, Dinges NG. Denver, CO, National Center for American Indian and Alaska Native Mental Health Research, 1988, pp 160–200

An excellent overview, this article provides data and expert discussion on the health status of the Indian elder and issues of concern to the field. Mental health is mentioned but is not a specific focus. Long-term care is discussed.

Conclusion

Although it has improved over the last decade, the literature on the Indian elder in general, and that relating to psychiatric illness in the Indian elderly in particular, remains sparse and frequently not published in mainstream journals. Much of the improvement may be credited to the work of Manson et al. at the National Center for American Indian/Alaska Native Mental Health Research in Denver. The work of the National Center places particular emphasis on mental health and long-term care issues. We are also seeing a few more published studies of particular disorders—notably depression—within this population.

In spite of this work, however, there remains a great need for studies of the Indian elderly in such areas as the epidemiology of mental disorder, the influence of culture on diagnosis, and treatment and patient management. Health services research into service use patterns of the Indian elderly would provide a more rational base for program planning. Existing data collected by the IHS provide little insight into these issues; improving IHS data collection must be a priority. Additionally, research activities must be broadened beyond the National Center in Denver.

In many cases, the psychiatric status of the Indian elderly appears to vary little from that of the majority elderly, but some research suggests that intriguing differences may be found in further study of the Indian elderly when compared with both other population groups of similar age and younger Indians. Such studies might demonstrate higher prevalence of some disorders than is found among the majority population, or they might demonstrate a lower prevalence, suggesting protective factors that might be identified and built upon. Clearly, one of the next key research steps is learning the risk factors for psychiatric disorders.

Such studies will have vast implications for the delivery of clinical services to the elderly American Indian population. Today, few services exist specifically for the Indian elderly, although some non-mental health programs, such as Alaska spirit camps, have implications for psychiatric service delivery.

Moreover, nonpsychiatric factors such as poverty and lack of transportation also affect psychiatric status. Although efforts to improve economic status and access to care are important, these should not be emphasized to the exclusion of clinical psychiatric care, as has often been the case in the past. Until the literature is vastly improved, psychiatric care of the Indian elderly will continue to be inadequate; it will continue to be based on ideology and "common knowledge" rather than on scientific fact. This is tragic in any population, but especially tragic in American Indian communities, in which the elder has always held an honored place.

Chapter 6

Issues in the Psychiatric Care of Asian/Pacific American Elders

Kenneth M. Sakauye, M.D.
Ranjit C. Chacko, M.D.

A 68-year-old Japanese-American woman sought treatment for chronic depression. She described herself as a *kibei*—American-born, but educated (through middle school) in Japan. Her parents had left Japan for the United States during the Meiji reform era (1868–1912) but sent her specifically to be educated in Japan. She was trapped in Japan during World War II and said she was teased mercilessly for being American. When she returned to the United States, she felt equally ostracized by the Japanese-American community, because she seemed "too Japanese." Throughout life, she continued to feel self-conscious and viewed herself as an outcast to both the non-Japanese and Japanese communities. She seemed to lack a firm sense of national or personal identity. Her main strength was that she was occupationally successful as a manager in a jewelry chain. However, she isolated herself socially to avoid further rejection or prejudicial behavior. The absence of recent experiences of prejudice served only as evidence for the success of her avoidant life-style. Although chronically depressed, the patient did not seek treatment until overwhelmed by the loss of her only close relationship (which was actually emotionally abusive). The patient showed strong, unresolved cultural conflicts resulting in lifelong identify problems, timidity, and extreme sensitivity to rejection and criticism.

Introduction

Between the 1980 and 1990 Census of Population and Housing, the Asian American population showed a 107.8% change, more than doubling its numbers to almost 7.3 million, largely due to heavy immigration from China, India, Korea, and the Phillipines in the 1980s. Seventeen separate Asian/Pacific Island ethnic groups are identified in the census: Chinese, Filipino, Japanese, Asian Indian, Korean, Vietnamese, Laotian, Thai, Cambodian, Pakistani, Indonesian, Hmong, Hawaiian, Samoan, Tongan, Guamanian, and Melanesian. However, approximately 84% of all Asian Americans residing in the United States are from six ethnic groups: Chinese, Filipino, Japanese, Korean, Vietnamese, and Asian Indian. Over 15% are Pacific Islanders. Due, in large part, to refugees and immigration, the median age of the overall Asian/Pacific Islander population is quite young—29.0 years. However, the percentage of elderly (over 62) ranges widely among Asian/Pacific Island ethnic groups: higher than the national average for Japanese (19.5%), similar to the national average for Chinese (12.5%) and Filipinos (now 11.3%), and much lower than the national average for Koreans (7.2%), Asian Indians (4.3%), and Vietnamese (4.6%). As a growing number of elderly individuals join families entering the United States in the most recent wave of immigration from Indochina, the number of newly immigrated elderly continues to rise.

The age disparity is partly explained by the effect of immigration laws toward Asians. The Asian Exclusion Act of 1917 barred admission to individuals east of an imaginary line drawn from the Red to the Mediterranean, Aegean, and Black seas; through the Caucasus Mountains and Caspian Sea; and along the Ural River and the Ural Mountains. This was repealed in stages beginning in 1943 (China) and later in 1946 (Phillipines) and 1952 (Japan and Korea), until all national quotas were lifted after 1965 (implemented 1968). The Indochinese Refugee Act, October 1977, allowed quota exceptions for these groups after 1978 and led to the Refugee Act of 1980, providing for a uniform admission procedure for refugees of all countries (based on the United Nations' definition of refugees; Chan 1983). The 1988 immigration amendments raised the worldwide ceiling of immigrants to a maximum of 590,000 (exclusion of refugees) and gave preference to family reunification (see Table 6–1).

The United States has experienced two distinct waves of Asian settle-

Table 6–1. Asian immigration patterns by country

Country	Decade totals					
	1891–1920	1921–1950[a]	1951–1960	1961–1970	1971–1980	1981–1990[b]
China	56,682	16,709	9,657	122,300	250,000	451,800
Japan	239,576	36,955	46,250	38,500	47,900	43,200
India	6,863	4,143	1,973	31,200	176,800	261,900
Korea	c	c	6,231	35,800	272,000	338,800
Philippines	c	c	19,307	101,500	360,200	495,300
Vietnam[d]	c	c	335	4,600	179,700	4,600
Cambodia[d]	c	c	—	1,200	8,400	116,60
Laos[d]	c	c	—	100	22,600	338,800
Thailand[d]	c	c	—	5,000	44,100	64,400
Other Asian countries[e]	20,660	32,161	92,226	1,307	1,538	3,023
Total, n	323,451	89,968	150,106	341,507	1,363,238	2,118,423
(mean/year)	(1,078)	(2,999)	(15,010)	(34,151)	(136,324)	(211,842)

[a]The Asian Exclusion Act of 1917 was sequentially repealed from 1943 to 1965.
[b]The Refugee Act of 1980 excluded groups defined as refugees by the United Nations from quota restrictions.
[c]Data not reported separately.
[d]The Indochinese Refugee Act of October 1977 excluded Indochinese refugees from quota restrictions.
[e]Other Asian countries prior to 1960 includes Asia and the Middle East.
Source. U.S. Immigration and Naturalization Service: *1987 Statistical Yearbook of the Immigration and Naturalization Service, National Series Data Program, 10/88.* Washington,DC, U.S. Department of Justice, 1988; United States Bureau of the Census: *Statistical Abstract of the United States, 1992,* 112th Edition. Washington, DC 1992; Chan S: *Asian Americans: An Interpretive History.* Boston, MA, Twayne Publishers, 1983.

ment. The first began with the opening of China and Japan to the West in the late 19th century and ended in 1917 when U.S. immigration laws banned Asian entry. The second wave began after 1943, when Asian immigration was sequentially liberalized. It peaked with the refugee assistance program in the late 1970s. Today's Asian elderly from the pre-1924 immigration wave are mainly American-born children of immigrants, although a few old-old immigrants are still alive. Asian elderly from the post-1943 immigrations are predominantly foreign born (see Table 6–2). However, even here, elderly differ with their temporal distance from immigration. The newest immigrant populations have large numbers of relatively new or poorly assimilated immigrants. Each group has different problems and needs.

Asian ethnic groups are highly diverse in culture and life-style. However, most articles on Asian/Pacific American mental health do not distinguish the study population by ethnicity, age, immigrant status, language competency, or social class. Almost no clinical literature exists on elderly Asian ethnic groups, with the exception of limited mental health studies of Japanese, Korean, and Chinese elderly.

Table 6–2.   Characteristics of Asian American elderly (age 65 and over) by ethnic group

			65 and older	
Ethnic group	Total population	Percentage 65 and over	Percentage foreign born	Median years of schooling
Chinese	812,178	10.8	75.9	6.8
Japanese	716,331	11.9	37.2	10.4
Korean	357,393	3.3	80.1	6.9
Filipino	781,894	13.3	96.3	7.5
Southeast Asian[a]	313,956	< 2[b]	100[b]	n/a
Asian Indian	387,223	15.7	19.3	11.2

[a]Subgroup populations for the Southeast Asian ethnic group are as follows: Cambodian, 16,044; Ethnic Chinese, n/a; Hmong, 5,204; Lao, 47,683; Mien, n/a; and Vietnamese, 245,025.
[b] Estimated.
Source.   Asian and Pacific Islander Population in the United States: 1980. 1980 Census of Population, Volume 2, Subject Reports (Issued January 1988).

A number of facts about the Asian American elderly are important for understanding their mental health status:

✦ Most Asian elderly are relatively recent immigrants (less than 10 years) of limited social and economic resources who face stress from culture shock.

✦ New immigrants or refugees, in general, are at highest risk for psychiatric problems such as adjustment disorders, depression, paranoia, and anxiety.

✦ The belief that Asian immigrants have a lower than average incidence of mental disorders is a misperception of service-use data. Low use rates most likely result not from an absence of mental health problems, but from financial or social barriers to care.

✦ High rates of economic assimilation are found among American-born Japanese and Asian American elderly; foreign-born minority elderly individuals from other Asian groups face multiple jeopardies similar to those faced by the African American and Hispanic elderly.

✦ Different culturally relevant issues apply to American born and immigrant Asian elderly. Professionals treating both immigrant and American-born Asian elderly should be aware of the cultural context of symptoms.

✦ Unanswered research questions remain about racial differences in metabolism, receptor density and sensitivity, rates of mental illness, validity of instruments and translations, prevalence of traditional beliefs and culture-bound syndromes, extent and nature of family conflicts, optimal treatment approaches, and appropriate cultural training for professionals and translators.

Diagnostic Issues

Culture-Bound Syndromes

Culture-bound syndromes such as *latah, amok, neurasthenia,* and other non-Western diagnoses have been described for Asians (see Table 6–3). These syndromes occur mainly in newly immigrated or unassimilated individuals, although rarely. Cultural belief systems usually explain such

Table 6–3.   Selected psychopathology and special health problems of Asians

Disorder	Prevalence
Genetic disorders[a]	
Alpha thalassemia carrier	3%–9% in Southeast Asians and Chinese Americans
Beta thalassemia carrier	5% in Southeast Asians and Chinese Americans
G-6-PD deficiency	4% rate in various Asian American groups
Lactose intolerance	> 50% estimates
Chronic health problems[b]	
Chronic hepatitis B	Highest in immigrants
Parasitism, tuberculosis	High in Southeast Asians
Cardiovascular mortality	Highest in Japanese (but less than the general population)
Cancer mortality	Higher gastrointestinal cancer rates
Cerebrovascular mortality	Highest in Japanese (compared with the general population)
Asians over 65 years who rate their health as poor	23% (Lin and Yu 1985)
Psychiatric syndromes[c]	
Depression	> 50% in new immigrants in a clinic setting
Suicide	High in Asian refugees
Shinkeishiusu	Japanese mixed neurotic picture
Anthropophobia	Japanese men; easy blushing and embarrassment
Latah	Southeast Asian women; exaggerated startle response to minimal stimuli
Amok	Southeast Asian men; sudden mass assault
Hwa byung	Korean, epigastric discomfort and morbid fear
Psychotropic medication differences[d]	
Tricyclic antidepressants	Efficacy at same dosage as whites; higher rates of side effects
Neuroleptics	Probably requires lower doses; higher rates of side effects at the same blood level of haloperidol
Benzodiazepines	Unknown

[a]Adapted from Office of Disease Prevention and Health Promotion: *Disease Prevention/Health Promotion: The Facts.* Washington, DC, U.S. Public Health Service, 1986.
[b]Adapted from Liu WT, Yu E: "Asian/Pacific American Elderly: Mortality Differentials, Health Status, and Use of Health Services." *J Appl Gerontol* 4:35–64, 1985; Stavig GR, Igra A, Leonard AR: "Hypertension and Related Health Issues Among Asians and Pacific Islanders in California." *Public Health Rep* 103:28–37, 1988.
[c]Adapted from Lin KM: "Hwa-Byung: A Korean Culture-Bound Syndrome?" *Am J Psychiatry* 140:105–107, 1983; Westermeyer J: "Psychiatric Diagnosis Across Cultural Boundaries." *Am J Psychiatry* 142:798–805, 1985; Bernstein RL, Gaw AC: "Koro: Proposed Classification for DSM-IV." 1990.
[d]No studies on the elderly. Inferences based on studies of younger adult Asians. World Health Organization: "Dose Effects of Antidepressant Medication in Different Populations: A World Health Organization Collaborative Study." *J Affect Disord* 2(suppl):S1–S67, 1986; Lin KM, Poland RE, Nakasaki G: *Psychopharmacology and Psychobiology of Ethnicity.* Washington, DC, American Psychiatric Press, 1993.

culture-bound syndromes as physical or organic illness, humoral imbalance (*yin/yang, am/duong*), or the result of malevolent spirits. Traditionally, the Confucian concept of mental illness does not involve either intrapsychic problems or learned behavior. However, traditional beliefs may not be widespread anymore, even in the countries of origin, because of contact with Western medicine and culture. It may be found predominantly among the elderly subgroups of each ethnic population. The extent of and adherence to cultural diagnoses and treatment approaches must be studied further because professional knowledge of cultural issues such as these are important in providing treatment to individuals who hold such beliefs.

Diagnostic Issues Bibliography

Westermeyer J: Psychiatric diagnosis across cultural boundaries. Am J Psychiatry 142:798–805, 1985

> The author presents a review of culture-bound syndromes including suicide (high in Asian refugees), *shinkeishiusu* (mixed neurosis found among Japanese), anthropophobia (easy blushing and embarrassment in Japanese men), *latah* (exaggerated startle response in Southeast Asian women), and *amok* (sudden mass assault among Southeast Asian men).

Lin KM: Hwa-byung: a Korean culture-bound syndrome? Am J Psychiatry 140:105–107, 1983

> Three cases of *hwa-byung,* a Korean folk illness designation for patients suffering from repressed or suppressed anger of long duration, are described. The illness manifests itself with various somatic symptoms. The main discomfort centers around the epigastrium and a morbid fear of impending death occurs. The author argues that somatization may be a culturally patterned method for Korean patients who are suffering from major depression to express their distress. The disorder is helped by antidepressant medication and supportive psychotherapy.

Health and Mortality Issues

The onset of chronic illness or disability is often a major precipitant of psychiatric problems for the elderly. Although overall Asians demonstrate better health than the general population, significant variations may exist across subgroups. For instance, life-style differences such as high salt content in traditional diets makes hypertension and multi-infarct dementia especially high risks for some groups. Prior environmental exposures of immigrants to parasitic infections, hepatitis, tuberculosis, or toxins may also be specially high risks for chronic disease states, especially in Southeast Asian and Chinese elderly. In addition, many genetic variants such as thalassemias, G-6-PD deficiency, and lactose intolerance are often present at higher frequencies than is usually suspected (see Table 6–3).

Suicide rates for elderly Asians—an indirect measure of mental illness or despair—have been difficult to interpret. Compared with age-matched data for the general population, the overall rate of suicide among Asians appears lower than the average, but this seems to vary by ethnic group and region and may be underreported. Risk factors for suicide and depression (isolation, poverty, and untreated posttraumatic stress disorders) are high in elderly refugees, although whether the sequelae of these risk factors include mental illness and suicide rates has not been established.

Racial differences in hepatic metabolism and other biological processes, as well as body size, may affect dose requirements for medications or other biological treatments for psychiatric disorders. Among the less-assimilated Asians, drugs may interact with herbal treatments or other traditional cures. Unfortunately, the few studies of differential pharmacokinetics among Asians do not discuss the elderly and, hence, are not cited in this review.

Health and Mortality Issues Bibliography

Group for the Advancement of Psychiatry (GAP), Committee on Cultural Psychiatry: Suicide and Ethnicity in the United States (Report No 128). New York, Brunner/Mazel, 1989

This monograph reviews both theories of and existing data on suicide by Hispanic Americans, African Americans, American Indians and

Alaska Natives, and Chinese and Japanese. Acculturation status poses an important missing variable in current data. Data on Asian ethnic groups is very limited, but Asian Americans who do commit suicide (irrespective of age), seem to be first-generation who speak no English, are of low socioeconomic status, and are unable to support themselves. Chinese and Japanese elderly have the highest suicide rates. The authors speculate that the departure of children from values of filial piety and respect are considered an ultimate rejection. On the assumption that acculturative stress is a major suicide risk factor for Asians, the authors postulate refugees (involuntary migrants) are at greatest risk. Voluntary and migrant immigrants have a somewhat lower risk, nonmigrant native groups an even lower risk, and nonmigrant established native groups the lowest risk.

Stavig GR, Igra A, Leonard AR: Hypertension and related health issues among Asians and Pacific Islanders in California. Public Health Rep 103:28–37, 1988

In this study, blood pressure measurements were taken on 8,353 adults living in California, of whom 1,757 were Asians and Pacific Islanders. More than 71% of the Asian group subjects were age 50 years or older. Subjects were asked six questions about awareness of hypertension and the risks of high blood pressure and their knowledge of methods for blood pressure control. The prevalence of hypertension in the Asians ages 50 and older differed widely among ethnic subgroups; pooled data showed 49.1% of men and 37.1% of women suffered from hypertension. More than 40% of the subjects had uncontrolled hypertension, and they were less likely to be aware of their hypertension than those individuals of other races with hypertension. The low treatment rate, low number of physician visits, and poor knowledge about hypertension may be related to a strong reliance on traditional healing. Moreover, Filipinos had high levels of poverty and low levels of education, further contributing to the knowledge deficit. The findings of this study suggest that Asians and Pacific Islanders may be at unusually high risk for hypertension-related problems such as multi-infarct dementia.

Office of Disease Prevention and Health Promotion: Disease Preven-
tion/Health Promotion: The Facts—U.S. Public Health Service. Palo
Alto, CA, Bull Publishing Co, 1986

Pooled data on the Asian elderly are presented, revealing remarkably
good life expectancies and health statuses. The health data did not
reflect differences related to being foreign-born or of low socioeconomic status (as the latter is seen in many newly immigrated Asian
subgroups). The major health risks for older Asians included 1) a
higher age-adjusted risk for stroke, 2) higher morbidity from diabetes,
3) higher risk of hypertension in some groups, and 4) high cholesterol
levels in some groups. Southeast Asians (all ages) had much higher
rates of the following: illness caused by intestinal parasites (61%),
positive tuberculosis test (55%), anemia (37%), hepatitis B antigen
(14%), and abnormal Venereal Disease Research Laboratory syphilis
test (12%). Compared with the general population, Asian minority
populations (all ages) had 1) lower death rates from suicide or homicide, 2) lower rates of smoking, 3) lower rates of alcoholism, and 4)
lower rates of obesity. Mental health data are largely unavailable, but
the article cites an unpublished study of Chinese Americans in New
York in which somatization disorders and major depression were
higher than in the general population in the 25–44 age group.

Liu WT, Yu E: Asian/Pacific American elderly: mortality differentials, health
status, and use of health services. J Appl Gerontol 4:35–64, 1985

This study examines data on Asian elderly individuals contained in
National Center for Health Statistics (NCHS) vital statistics records
and special health surveys—the National Health Interview Survey, the
National Health and Nutrition Examination Survey, and the National
Ambulatory Medical Survey. A number of interesting findings in important areas were uncovered. Regarding economic status, for instance, counter to the belief that all Asian Americans are financially
comfortable, Chinese, Japanese, and Filipinos were reported to earn
consistently less than whites. A large number of Asian subgroups were
worse off than the general population on both social and economic
characteristics. Regarding mortality, among Chinese, Japanese, and

Filipino Americans, it was lower than among white Americans in every age group. Lower than average percentages of these minority groups rated their health as poor. (Data on other Asian American subgroups are absent from the NCHS files.) Foreign-born death rates exceeded native-born rates by two to five times in the age groups reported. Three studies are cited that suggest cancer death rates were highest in the first generation. Regarding number of medical visits, little difference was found in visits to physicians and dentists by Asian Americans; however, hospital stays were longer than for any other ethnic group, suggesting more serious illnesses among Asian Americans. Regarding differences between foreign-born and native-born elderly, data were limited. Asian immigrants appeared to avoid all but emergency medical help from other than traditional healers and methods. Regarding health insurance, overall medical insurance subscription rates were low among Asian elderly, posing a major barrier to care.

Peterson MR, Rose CL, McGee RI: A cross-cultural health study of Japanese and Caucasian Asians in Hawaii. Int J Aging Hum Dev 21:267–279, 1985

A study of Hawaii State Department of Health data files of 1,098 Japanese and 873 whites ages 60 and over reveals that better health was predicted, not only by younger age, higher family income, and maintenance of work role, but also by Japanese ethnicity per se. The authors suggest that the monolithic doctrine of disadvantaged status of minority groups may need to be reconsidered for some ethnic groups.

McIntosh JL, Santos JF: Suicide among minority elderly: a preliminary investigation. Suicide Life Threat Behav 11:151–166, 1981

This report, based on 1976 cause-of-death summary tapes from the National Center for Health Statistics, focuses on suicide among elderly Native Americans, African Americans, Japanese Americans, Chinese Americans, and Filipino Americans. Suicide rates had been increasing for nonwhites; the rates also were increasing with age. Although the rates were generally very low for the majority of minority aged, the suicide rates among elderly Chinese (23.07 per 100,000) and Japanese

(22.51 per 100,000) were higher than that among whites (21.02 per 100,000). Higher suicide rates in these two populations, the authors postulate, may reflect cultural acceptance of suicide as a coping mechanism. Low levels in African American and Indian groups are thought to be a product of both survivor status (i.e., only the fittest with the most resiliency can survive) and the presence of buffers from social importance and role.

Valle R: Natural support systems, minority groups, and the late life dementias: implications for service delivery, research, and policy, in Clinical Aspects of Alzheimer's Disease and Senile Dementia (Aging, Vol 15). Edited by Miller NE, Cohen GD. New York, Raven, 1981, pp 277–299

Studies of minority group elderly support networks and behavior problems are largely impressionistic and often lack empirical validation. The author discusses the clinical interface among minority elderly, natural support systems, and formal services at different stages of disability. No data had been amassed to detail the incidence or prevalence of later life dementia among minority groups. However, the existing literature suggested the following for minority elderly: 1) Deleterious life conditions may make the presence of dementias more significant in young-old minority patients; 2) Lower rates of morbidity among the oldest-old may be due to crossover effects (only the fittest survive to extended old age, so old-old minority individuals are actually healthier than their white counterparts); 3) Underclass status and multiple jeopardy limit access to health care, so resource use may be reserved for the more catastrophic or advanced stages of illness; and 4) The increasing numbers and longevity of minority elderly will affect rates of service use.

Ibrahim IB, Carter C, McLaughlin D, et al: Ethnicity and suicide in Hawaii. Soc Biol 24:10–16, 1977

Three racial groups were selected for study: Japanese, whites, and Filipinos. Japanese exhibited the highest tendency to commit suicide, and Filipinos exhibited the least. Among Japanese, the incidence of suicide rose proportionally with age; among whites and Filipinos, the risk had an inverse relationship to age. However, trends suggested figures were approaching a common value.

Kalish RA: Suicide: an ethnic comparison in Hawaii. Bulletin of Suicidology 4:37–43, 1968

Honolulu Department of Health suicide data from 1959 to 1965 were analyzed by ethnicity, sex, and age, and compared with general indexes of social disorganization (e.g., crime, divorce, and psychiatric hospital-ization rates). Suicide rates among Koreans, Japanese, and Chinese appeared to increase with age. The study also found that suicide rates rose concomitantly with occupational class.

Presentation of Psychiatric Disorders

Communication of Illness

The language patients use to describe affective concerns is often difficult to translate. In Asian cultures, for example, the Confucian value placed on stoicism and self-sacrifice has yielded Minnesota Multiphasic Personality Inventory patterns of depression or schizoid tendencies, by U.S. standards, within normal individuals. An older Asian patient may not see the rele-vance of verbatim translations of certain items from standard mental health questionnaires. For example, "feeling blue" and "feeling guilty" are not typical Asian complaints in depression. The Japanese term for depres-sion, *yuutsu,* uses nature metaphors (rain, storm, dark, mountains) as descriptors. Neither the sensitivity nor the specificity of translated versions of diagnostic questionnaires that are intended to disclose specific mental disorders has been established for the Asian elderly. Few bilingual Asian professionals or professional translators are available, making language barriers a potential cause of misdiagnoses or missed diagnoses in non-English speaking individuals.

Communication of Illness Bibliography

Marsella AJ, Kameoka VA: Ethnocultural issues in the assessment of psy-chopathology, in Measuring Mental Illness: Psychometric Assessment for Clinicians. Edited by Wetzler S. Washington, DC, American Psychiatric Press, 1989, pp 229–256

The authors present four evaluative components of cross-cultural assessment for which, ideally, cultural equivalence should be established: language, concepts, scales, and norms. A methodological discussion comparing existing scales and indigenous assessment tools follows. Examples are provided of when cultural influences may lead to misdiagnoses. Concepts such as dependency, depression, anxiety, aggression, anger, jealousy, death, love, suicide, and person are not equivalent across cultures. The authors note that the American Psychological Association Code of Ethics urges that clinicians be trained in cultural knowledge and awareness before engaging in clinical activities with patients from different cultural groups.

Hughes GW: Neuropsychiatric aspects of bilingualism: a brief review. Br J Psychiatry 139:25–28, 1981

Differential language loss or recovery in multilingual patients who become aphasic is a generally accepted phenomenon. Differential language loss in other bilinguals is also observed in which the second language is forgotten first. However, functional preferences (e.g., hallucinatory voices in one language only, or affective connotations in one language only) may not fit this pattern. The review implies that possible compartmentalization of thought processes by language may complicate treatment of bilingual or multilingual patients.

Prevalence of Psychiatric Disorders

Pilot studies on the mental health of the Asian elderly show low rates of psychopathology in most Asian populations. However, samples are small and do not represent the diversity that exists within the ethnic groups. There are older studies of non-Asian immigrants, such as the Midtown Manhattan Study (Srole et al. 1962), that demonstrated there are high rates of mental health problems in the early adjustment years for immigrants of all ages.

Prevalence of Psychiatric Disorders Bibliography

Biser M: Influences of time, ethnicity, and attachment on depression in Southeast Asian refugees. Am J Psychiatry 145:46–51, 1988

The study investigates whether certain phases of resettlement are accompanied by an elevated risk for depression among Southeast Asian refugees in Canada. Sex and age did not contribute to an increased risk of psychopathology in this study. However, the number of elderly in the sample was not reported. In general, the longer the refugees remained in Canada, the better their mental health status. Unmarried or otherwise single Laotians and Vietnamese refugees experienced the highest levels of depression within 10–12 months after arrival. Two years after the initial investigation, the socially disadvantaged group (unmarried, unattached) remained more depressed than other refugee groups.

Yamamoto J, Yamamoto M, Steinberg A, et al: Alcohol abuse among elderly Asians in Los Angeles: a pilot study. Pacific/Asian American Mental Health Research Center Research Review 6:26–27, 1988

Interview data using the Diagnostic Interview Schedule (Version III) were reported for Chinese, Japanese, and Filipinos ages 65 and older. Whereas the rates of alcoholism for all three groups were lower than that found in the general population, they were intermediate in cross-cultural comparisons with the countries of origin. The authors suggest that as Asians become more acculturated, the sociocultural protection against drinking problems will be lost and drinking patterns will more closely resemble those of the United States generally.

Hayes CL: Two worlds in conflict: the elderly Hmong in the United States, in Ethnic Dimensions of Aging. Edited by Gelfand DE, Barresi CM. New York, Springer, 1987, pp 79–95

Open-ended, in-depth interviews of 19 Hmong elderly (ages 40–78) were conducted to explore adjustment following immigration to the United States. Compared with Vietnamese and Cambodian refugees,

Laotians (including the Hmong) are technologically undeveloped. The Hmong had few skills other than farming. Interviewees stressed problems arising from altered family structures (including the absence of work). They often emphasized themes of loss—of possessions, mobility, religious customs, and status. Depression was denied but may actually be present. Community informants stated that 90% of elders complained of poor sleep, poor appetite, prolonged sadness, and agitation. The informants noted that many elderly appeared to live in the past, or cried continually. None of those interviewed had received mental health assistance. Families seemed uncertain how to handle elders with mental health problems.

Yamamoto J, Machizawa S, Araki F, et al: Mental health of elderly Asian Americans in Los Angeles. American Journal of Social Psychiatry 5:37–46, 1985

The authors review the history and current status of psychiatric epidemiology in the United States and Asia and discuss methodological difficulties inherent in community surveys. This pilot survey in Los Angeles used the Diagnostic Interview Schedule (Versions II and III on different waves of subjects) to evaluate 122 primarily elderly subjects from Japanese community service programs and a Japanese home for the aged. High rates of psychiatric disorders were found in both samples. In the community sample, 60% evidenced some symptoms of somatization disorder, 27% dysthymic disorder, 3% major depressive disorder, and 10% schizophrenic disorder. High rates of organic brain syndrome (45%) were found in the community sample. The nursing home group had higher rates of dysthymia and lower rates of somatization and schizophrenia, and a surprisingly lower degree of organic brain syndrome. The data counter the stereotype that the Japanese elderly have few mental health problems, and highlight the need for special consideration for services. (*Note.* The authors, in a personal communication, stated that data on 100 Korean elderly are being collected.)

Yu E, Liu WT, Kurzeja P: Physical and mental health status indicators for Asian/Pacific Americans—Subreport prepared for the Report of the

Secretary's Task Force on Black and Minority Health. Washington, DC, U.S. Government Printing Office, 1985

Existing studies with recommendations are summarized.

Kuo WH: Prevalence of depression among Asian-Americans. J Nerv Ment Dis 172:449–457, 1984

The dearth of population-based studies and epidemiologic investigations of psychiatric disorders among Asian Americans has led to contradictory speculations about the prevalence rates of mental illness in this population. This investigation compared Center for Epidemiologic Studies–Depression Scale scores of 499 Chinese, Filipinos, Japanese, and Koreans with those of whites and other minority groups. The results for those age 60 or older showed that Korean elderly immigrants scored higher on depression than whites or other Asian groups, and that, as a whole, Asian Americans scored higher than their white counterparts. Evidence also suggested higher numbers of somatic complaints accompanying depressive complaints among the Asian American population.

Liu WT, Lamanna M, Murata A: Transition to Nowhere: Vietnamese Refugees in America. Nashville, TN, Charter House, 1979

The study was based on interviews of refugees at Camp Pendleton in 1975. Only 5 of 202 respondents were age 65 or over. The extent of mental illness and the determination not to seek treatment was high among all age groups. However, the older individuals appeared to be in the best spirits and able to handle their responsibility for family chores. Younger heads of household, in contrast, seemed to manifest the greatest futility, homesickness, and depression. Sorrow and grief were viewed as natural, and cultural inhibitions seemed to preclude expression of psychological issues.

Rahe RH, Looney JG, Ward HW, et al: Psychiatric consultation in a Vietnamese refugee camp. Am J Psychiatry 135:185–190, 1978

The authors provided psychiatric consultation to a Vietnamese refugee camp in California. The Recent Life Changes Questionnaire, Cornell Medical Index-Health Questionnaire, and Self-Anchoring Scale (of how close or far an individual was from his worst or best possible world) were given to 200 randomly selected refugees. Some subjects were age 50 or older. Refugees in all age groups showed moderately high psychological symptoms and low morale; the oldest groups showed the highest number of mental health complaints. The greatest number of elderly expressed the sense that they were in the worst of their imagined worlds.

Family and Support Issues

The family network serves as a major buffer against stress. Unfortunately, family support is often inadequate or absent for many Asian elderly individuals. For example, many elderly Chinese immigrated decades ago without family, and new immigrant families are often separated. Even in intact families, the stereotype of Asian family closeness may be misleading. A strong sense of filial responsibility may exist, but feelings of closeness may be low. The emphasis on assimilation for younger members of the family magnifies polarities between the new and traditional values or life-styles and intensifies intergenerational conflicts. Some reports suggest that intergenerational conflict is most marked within the first three generations after immigration. To date, no systematic study has been undertaken to examine the extent or the impact of intergenerational conflicts in Asian minority families.

Family and Support Issues Bibliography

Sakauye KM: Ethnic variations in family support of the frail elderly, in Family Involvement in Treatment of the Frail Elderly. Edited by Zucker-Goldstein M. Washington, DC, American Psychiatric Press, 1989, pp 63–106

The author reviews the literature in this area and reports that caregiving seems to begin earlier in the family cycle for low socioeconomic status minority groups. Immigrant status often heightens inter-generational conflicts; psychiatric comorbidity with physical illness seems especially high. Lower service use may be related to stigma or to fears of high cost and inadequate services rather than a cultural bias. Based on the data, the needs for outreach, patient education, and services linked to medical care appear to be the most pressing.

Osako MM: Japanese Americans: melting into the all-American pot? in Ethnic Chicago. Edited by Jones d'A, Hilli MG. Grand Rapids, MI, Eerdmans, 1983, pp 314–344

The author presents a microsocial view of the processes of adjustment, survival, and identity change of the Japanese in the Midwest. The impact of internment of Issei men (elderly immigrant generation) was reported to be the most severe life trauma that undermined the fabric of the Japanese community and family. Speculations on the long-term psychological impact of this event are made, but data are absent.

Nandi PK: The Quality of Life of Asian Americans: An Exploratory Study in a Middle-Size Community. Chicago, IL, Pacific-American Mental Health Resource Center, 1980

Forty-five in-depth, open-ended, tape-recorded interviews were con-ducted with a small but representative sample of Indians, Pakistanis, Chinese, Filipinos, and Koreans living in midsize communities that, by and large, had not been included in prior sociological inquiries. Like the general community, the sample was not economically disadvan-taged. Six of the subjects were between ages 51 and 60; no subjects were over 61. The author comments on the high sense of displacement, loss of position, and nonveneration of the oldest group. Depression, anxi-ety, and mental illness were not assessed.

Wu F: Mandarin-speaking aged Chinese in the Los Angeles area. Gerontol-ogist 15:271–275, 1975

For centuries, care of the aged was not a major social problem in China; the Confucian teaching—the Hsiao Ching of family responsibility—was deeply ingrained in the Chinese culture. This Los Angeles study found that Mandarin-speaking elderly struggle with political, social, economic, and cultural changes, including changes in the precept of filial piety. The inability to speak or understand English has been the most serious problem among elderly who had immigrated in old age. Language barriers and cultural shock alienate the Chinese elderly from mainstream American society and exclude them from needed services.

Chen P: A study of Chinese American elderly residing in hotel rooms. Soc Casework 60:89–95, 1979

A study of elderly Chinese American residents in the Chinatown area of Los Angeles reveals hidden poverty, loneliness, language barriers, physical isolation, a sense of familial dislocation, and a lack of concern for the future. Work is suggested to develop programs and services to meet the needs of this population.

Nahirny VC, Fishman JA: American immigrant groups: ethnic identification and the problem of generations. Sociol Rev 13:311–326, 1965

This article presents observations on the patterns of intergenerational conflict associated with the course of assimilation, most noticeably occurring within three generations. The author describes the first American-born generation as feeling some cultural shame—shame for their parents, downplaying their ethnic heritage. Their children, in turn, wish to revive the ethnic heritage, of which they have little knowledge. The use of the ethnic mother tongue usually ends by the third generation. This model helps explain generation gaps, but provides no confirming data.

Barriers to Care

The high prevalence of immigrant elderly individuals in the Asian population creates the need for bilingual and ethnically identified programs to meet their mental health and other needs. The low use of nursing homes and elderly housing by the Asian elderly may be due to the absence of ethnically identified services. Asian community groups in many major cities have responded to the dearth of service programs by building and using their own Asian elderly housing and nursing homes. Thus, when facilities are accepted by the ethnic group, resistance to the use of formal services is virtually eliminated.

Other reasons for low use by Asian elderly are comparable to those identified in other minority elderly populations: lack of knowledge about services, financial barriers, language barriers, and preference for traditional care for some disorders. The fear of prejudicial treatment is a factor for Asians as for any minority ethnic group.

Barriers to Care Bibliography

Braun KL, Humphrey JW, Kaku JM: Community long-term care for geriatric patients in Hawaii. Hawaii Med J 46:417–431, 1987

The authors evaluated use of and preference for four long-term care options among ethnic elderly groups (Japanese, Filipino, Chinese, Hawaiian, white) on Oahu. The Japanese constitute a majority of day-hospital patients, whites heavily use nursing homes and foster-family programs, and Filipinos show a predilection for foster care. Although outpatient-program patients generally were more cognitively intact and had fewer problems with incontinence, these factors did not fully account for relative preferences for outpatient services.

Hing E: Use of nursing homes by the elderly: preliminary data from the 1985 nursing home survey (DHHS Publ No PHS-87-1250), Advance Data from Vital and Health Statistics No 135. Hyattsville, MD, Public Health Service, 1987

Racial differences in long-term-care use were seen in the 1985 National Nursing Home Survey. Whites showed a rate of 47.6 per 1,000, African Americans showed a rate of 35.0 per 1,000, and other races showed a rate of 20.1 per 1,000. The data suggest a need to analyze preferences of, and alternative care mechanisms sought for, elderly individuals in minority populations.

Cox C: Physician utilization by three groups of ethnic elderly. Med Care 24:667–676, 1986

Determinants of physician use were examined among three groups of ethnic elderly individuals living in Santa Clara, California—Vietnamese, Portuguese, and Hispanic. Structured personal interviews about physician use were administered to 100 members of each ethnic group over age 60. Among the Vietnamese, satisfaction with medical care was the most significant predictor of use. Language of the physician was also an important predictor. Attitudes about psychiatric care were not included in the study protocol.

Liu WT: Health services for Asian elderly. Res Aging 8:156–175, 1986

Data show that not all elderly Asians are cared for by kin or by their ethnic community. The article points out the dearth of systematic knowledge of patterns of health service use among Asian American elderly.

Matsushima NM, Tashima N: Mental Health Treatment Modalities of Pacific/Asian American Practitioners (NIMH Grant 1-RO1 MH32148), A Report of the Pacific Asian Mental Health Research Project. San Francisco, CA, 1982

A survey of Asian/Pacific American practitioners was conducted on 715 individuals of Asian surname who had been listed in professional directories. Fifty-four of the questionnaires were returned uncompleted, because the practitioners said they either did not work with Asian/Pacific patients or were no longer in practice. Of the 347 practitioners who replied (50% social workers, 11% psychiatrists, 16% psychologists, 14% paraprofessionals, and 10% in other professions), Southeast Asian respondents maintained the highest proportion of Asian/Pacific Islanders in their case loads (91%); such practitioners generally were nonpsychiatrists. Only 53% of respondents used languages other than English in their practices, and 41% had less than 25% Asians in their practice. Almost 8% of the sample used supplemental indigenous treatment modalities in their practice.

Moon A, Tashima N: Help-seeking Behavior and Attitudes of Southeast Asian Refugees (Funded by NIMH Grant No 1-RO1 MH32148). San Francisco, CA, Pacific Asian Mental Health Research Project, 1982

Randomly selected individuals ($N = 396$) from the six major Indochinese groups (Cambodian, Hmong, ethnic Chinese, Lao, Mien, and Vietnamese) were interviewed. Ages ranged from 18 to 81, with a median age of 34.6 years. Although 25% of the interview subjects were over age 40, data for the elderly were not analyzed separately. Interview subjects indicated little use of external formal supports or services for symptoms of mental or emotional problems; however, they would readily use medical services for physical illness. Many social problems (homesickness, loneliness, nutrition) were listed as major concerns. Most interviewees considered the use of external mental health professionals to be a last resort. Cost and location did not appear to influence this decision. Moreover, the family also played a less important role than expected. Local healers and healing practices appeared to be the first line of treatment. The survey suggests that confidence in the provider must be built (by language, cultural sensitivity, and community involvement) before services will be used.

Fujii SM: Elderly Asian Americans and use of public services. Soc Casework 57:202–207, 1976

Cultural differences have hindered Asian immigrant adjustment to the dominant society. The author describes information presented at the 1971 White House Conference on Aging addressing the low rates of use of public services by the Asian elderly. She fears racism and cultural barriers continue beyond the immigrant generation and advocates special programs for Asian American elderly.

Kitano HL: Japanese-American mental illness, in Changing Perspectives in Mental Illness. Edited by Plog S, Edgerton R. New York, Holt, Rinehart & Winston, 1969, pp 256–284

Factors causing low use rates for psychiatric services among Japanese Americans include cost, existing support mechanisms, misdiagnosis or labeling problems, negative attitudes toward mental health care by the Japanese, higher rates of family care, and a "lack of a mentally ill role." The author notes that acculturation is altering these factors over time, and that the "older ways of treatment through the family, extended family, and community will soon give way to the use of professionals, of experts, and of institutions."

Unique Concerns

New Immigrants

New immigrants suffer multiple jeopardies: culture shock, difficulty learning a second language, decreased value for their cultural knowledge or experience, fewer opportunities for education or occupational involvement, and greater social alienation. Newly immigrated elderly face a high risk for mental illness.

Bilingual, ethnic professionals appear to be needed to work with newly immigrated elderly or those who have not learned English. Use of translators is limiting: translators may be inexperienced, the dialogue stilted as the result of the translation process; patients may communicate selectively if family or friends serve as translators. Moreover, bilingual, ethnic professionals may share with the patient a common understanding of attitudes and nonverbal communications. In fact, a survey of Asian American practitioners revealed that bilingual professionals often use Eastern healing approaches that are not taught in the Unites States in combination with "Western" therapies with Asian patients (see Table 6–4).

New Immigrants Bibliography

Gozdiak E: What providers need to know to serve older refugees. The Aging Connection (The American Society on Aging newsletter), April/May, 1990, pp 7, 10

This article highlights some of the sources of strain for aged refugees resettled in the United States. The strain of exile takes a physical toll, reflected in high rates of somatic complaints. The inability to converse in English diminishes further the elders' positions of authority and wisdom. Separated from their ancestors and ancestral homelands, many elderly refugees fear their own thoughts of death. Service delivery is difficult. Most aged refugees know little about available treatment opportunities. Moreover, such services are often far away from the refugees and lack bilingual or bicultural staff or others with an awareness of how to reach out to these refugees. The author emphasizes the importance of language and acculturation programs to teach refugees survival skills and literacy.

Weinstein-Shr G: Breaking the Linguistic and Social Isolation of Refugee Elders: An Intergenerational Model. (personal communication, 1988)

The Learning English through Intergenerational Friendship (LEIF) project at Temple University (Philadelphia, Pennsylvania) uses volunteer tutors to teach English in the homes of elderly refugees. Typically, an elderly refugee spends most of the time in the home caring for the small children; isolation is common. A case report on the isolation-related suicide of an elderly widowed Hmong woman highlights the

---

Table 6–4.   Selected mental health modalities used by Asian American practitioners with Asians

---

Ethnic mental health professionals: client-value orientations
  Pharmacotherapy
  Cognitive Behavioral
  Psychodynamic
  Phenomenological
  "Traditional + Western"

Eastern approaches used (not taught in the United States)
  Acupuncture
  Herbal medicine
  Morita therapy
  Naikan therapy
  Spiritual therapy
  Others

Source.   Adapted from Matsushima NM, Tashima N: *Mental Health Treatment Modalities of Pacific/Asian American Practitioners (NIMH Grant No 1-RO1 MH32148), A Report of the Pacific Asian Mental Health Research Project.* San Francisco, CA, 1982

need for community outreach. The program is predicated on the belief that uprooted elders will cope better if they have information about social services and have language skills to access them. The question of accessibility and acceptance by the refugee elders is not addressed.

Kuo WH: Social networking, hardiness, and immigrant's mental health. J Health Soc Behav 27:133–149, 1986

Previous investigations of immigrant hospitalization rates for mental disorders have accumulated inconclusive evidence regarding native-foreign differences. The author hypothesizes that immigrants are not solely reactive to stressful life changes. Rather, the chief means of ameliorating strain are the immigrant's activism in cultivating social networks and hardiness of personality. Immigration in older age, unfortunately, may preclude the development of such protective or adaptive mechanisms.

Kiefer CW, Kim S, Choi K, et al: Adjustment problems of Korean American elderly. Gerontologist 24:477–482, 1985

Fifty elderly Korean immigrants were intensively interviewed to identify typical adjustment problems in this group. Ratings of stress and adjustment were made in five areas of functioning: social, cultural, economic, physical, and emotional/cognitive. Adjustment was positively related to education, length of residence in the United States, and multigenerational household structure. As many earlier studies referenced in the article suggest, immigration, particularly from a non-Western culture, is usually stressful, with serious psychological effects for some years after the event itself. The situation is complicated further when the immigrant cannot be absorbed into a large, well-established ethnic community. The authors help identify older immigrants who are at special risk for poor adaptation and argue that services should be targeted to these elderly.

Koh S, Sakauye KM, Koh TH, et al: A reflection on the study of Asian American elderly by Asian American researchers. Asian American Psychological Association Journal 8:22–33, 1983

Limitations in achieving the goals of the model project for Asian American elderly (initially described in Koh et al. 1981) were discussed. The highest-risk individuals (newest isolated immigrants) could not be recruited. Most subjects had had prestudy involvement in church or other Korean organizations, had been in the United States for several years, and had demonstrated good premorbid psychological adjustment. Even limited conversational English was never achieved by the study subjects despite intensive English as a second language training, pointing out a need for further psycholinguistic studies of the elderly. Experiential insights into the nature of culturally sensitive research and a critique of scales are discussed.

Koh S, Sakauye KM, Koh TH: Adaptive capabilities of newly immigrated Asian elderly. Quarterly Contact 4:3, 1981

The authors describe a model intervention program for newly immigrated Korean elderly individuals that provides a "survival English" course; orientation to the new social customs; and peer support in a 6-month, informal, group-learning setting. Korean elderly individuals who immigrated to reunite with their children were thought to be at a particularly high risk for adjustment problems, because Korean families have geographically dispersed residence patterns, and because the elderly are isolated from both the Korean community and the work force. In addition, immigrant elderly individuals show problems in new-language acquisition and in obtaining information about leisure activities, both of which make adjustment difficult.

Lin KM, Tazuma L, Masuda M: Adaptational problems of Vietnamese refugees; I: health and mental health status. Arch Gen Psychiatry 36:955–961, 1979

Masuda M, Lin KM, Tazuma L: Adaptational problems of Vietnamese Refugees; II: life changes and perception of life events. Arch Gen Psychiatry 37:447–450, 1980

The authors report in two parts on a 2-year study of Vietnamese refugees on whom the Cornell Medical Index was administered in

1975 and again in 1976. The results indicated a high and continuing level of physical and mental dysfunction in over 50% of the sample. Clinically, many Vietnamese suffered from psychosomatic symptoms, depression, and anxiety. The oldest subpopulation (ages 47 and older) represented 15% of the original sample. Higher impairment was seen with increasing age.

Kuo W: Theories of migration and mental health: an empirical testing on Chinese-Americans. Soc Sci Med 10:297–306, 1976

This study tested the applicability of four theoretically most stressful life-change components for new immigrants that are related to mental health. The four theoretical components—social isolation, culture shock, goal-striving stress, and cultural change were explicated and tested against a data set of 170 Chinese immigrants residing in the Washington, D.C., area. The four items accounted for less than 25% of the variance of the mental impairment scores (General Well-Being; Midtown Psychiatric Impairment Index, used in the Midtown Manhattan study, and the Center for Epidemiologic Studies–Depression Scale, or CES-D). The study demonstrates that the impact of immigration is highly complex, and the major stressors have not been clearly outlined.

Sauna VD: Immigration and mental illness: a review of the literature with special emphasis on schizophrenia, in Behavior in New Environments. Edited by Brody E. Beverly Hills, CA, Sage, 1969, pp 291–352

This article reviews 88 studies relating immigration to mental illness. Almost none of the studies controlled for age or compared the migrant population to the home country to determine cohort effects. A meta-analysis of these studies was not undertaken. The author notes extreme variability in study results, reflecting the complex interactions among age, sex, education, social class, and other variables. He also posits that the studies are affected by sampling bias, because they depend upon service use statistics as the primary measure of pathology. The primary causes of the variable results across studies include 1) the motivation for migration, 2) the type of environment in which the migrant previously resided, and 3) the personal characteristics of the migrant. The author notes that no evidence supports the once-prevailing theory that immigrants were likely to have mental illness because they were "defectives" who were being "dumped" by their mother countries.

U.S.-Born Asian Elderly

U.S.-born Asian Americans (predominantly Asian Indian and Japanese) generally have achieved good economic assimilation, though most have confronted prejudicial attitudes and barriers in their lifetimes. Despite a progressive loss of cultural knowledge and language from generation to generation, and less adherence to traditional values, a sense of ethnic identification is generally maintained, and the majority of Asian American elderly individuals still maintain membership in an ethnic organization (church, association, or club). The effects of prejudice and exclusion may also have long-term psychological consequences—neurotic symptoms or lost self-esteem—although the prevalence of more severe psychiatric disorders is probably no higher than is found in the general population. Case studies and reports have detailed passivity, reduced aspirations, delayed marriage, fewer numbers of children, and self-esteem difficulties as common "traits" that are not seen in the countries of origin.

U.S.-Born Asian Elderly Bibliography

Yamamoto J, Wagatsuma H: The Japanese and Japanese Americans. Journal of Operational Psychiatry 11:120–1335, 1980

Two studies are presented to highlight the positive effect of "cultural buffering." Cultural values and acculturation experiences seem to exert a strong effect on affiliative preferences and behaviors. The article describes attitudes about the mother-child relationship, individualism (*kojinshugi*), selfishness, and community relations (*rko-shugi*), and the group trauma of encampment during World War II. The impact of acculturation difficulties was inferred from suicide rates (higher than among the general U.S. population), divorce rates (between those of Japan and the United States), crime rates (between those of Japan and the United States), and mental disorders, based on inpatient hospitalization rates (between Japan's low rate and the United States' high rate). A sense of group cohesion, and a greater exposure to Japanese culture during upbringing, seemed to reduce stress-related disorders, including coronary heart disease, in this sample.

Babcock CG, Gehrie MJ: Psychoanalysis and follow-up: the personal and cultural meaning of the experience of Nisei in treatment (NIMH Fellowship Grant No 5-F22-MH02492-01,02 03). Paper presented at the Research Meeting of the Chicago Institute for Psychoanalysis, March 24, 1977

This long-term study, initiated in 1944 by a number of social scientists including Charlotte Babcock, Setsuko Nishi, Ruth Benedict, Margaret Mead, Talcott Parsons, Thomas French, Erich Lindemann, and Sol Ginsberg, attempted to understand and manage the psychological consequences of internment and prejudice. Fifty case studies of Japanese Americans who sought psychotherapy through the project (four in full psychoanalyses) were collected. This article presents an in-depth case summary of one Nisei's psychoanalysis and the 26-year follow-up at age 52. Enduring themes included anger about prejudice, unresolved differences with parents (who were seen as representing the "Japanese world"), defensive distancing in relationships, stoicism (enduring in silence), being identified as "acting like a Japanese," and continuing narcissistic vulnerability related to Japanese identity. There was no evidence of major psychiatric disturbance, although one could see areas of potential emotional vulnerability. Similar themes were reportedly found in the other study cases.

Supplying Special Programs

Special programs are needed to help new elderly immigrants reduce culture shock and isolation. Standard English as a second language programs are too seldom used by the elderly, in part due to teaching style or rapid pacing. Appropriately targeted language programs and health promotion programs directed specifically toward the elderly Asian immigrant may help reduce risk factors for depression.

Moreover, responses received by this task force from practitioners engaged in treating Asian/Pacific Americans emphasize a range of needs not currently or fully addressed in the care of the Asian elderly:

✦ Bilingual services
✦ Bicultural services that respect culturally disparate views of mental illness and intervention methods
✦ Race and age appropriate dose: response curves
✦ Outreach involving greater collaboration with the community's gate-keepers and social institutions
✦ Culturally sensitive scales, including scales that are sensitive to linguistic equivalents for depression and anxiety
✦ Efforts to address barriers restricting access to quality care
✦ Cultural psychiatry training for all professionals working with both American-born or immigrant Asian elderly

Supplying Special Programs Bibliography

Lin TY, Lin MC: Service delivery issues in Asian-North American communities. Am J Psychiatry 135:454–456, 1978

The authors cite sociocultural factors (moralistic, religious, psychological, and familial) that influence the help-seeking behavior of Chinese psychiatric patients in North America. They propose an approach for socioculturally relevant service delivery to Chinese. The main tenets involve locating services within the community, involving the local community leaders and social institutions, and maintaining a physician on the multidisciplinary treatment team, because physicians are still accorded special respect. Other canons are provision of a culturally relevant training program, use of bilingual workers who respect the Chinese view of mental illness and intervention methods, and exercise of special caution in prescribing psychotropic medication.

Sata LS: A profile of Asian-American psychiatrists. Am J Psychiatry 135:448–454, 1978

Of 367 respondents to a survey of Asian American members of the American Psychiatric Association, less than 16% were American-born

U.S. medical school graduates. Forty-one percent of the patients treated by the Asian American psychiatrists were minority group members. Asian psychiatrists had recently emerged as the largest visible multiethnic minority group in American psychiatry. Training programs for Asians, as for all other foreign medical school students, must provide opportunities to work through cultural differences and must support the significance of biculturalism and bilingual skills.

Uba L: Meeting the mental health needs of Asian Americans: mainstream or segregated services. Professional Psychology 12:215–221, 1982

This article presents current barriers to the use of mental health services by Asian Americans and discusses the advantages and disadvantages of three prototypes of culturally sensitive service delivery systems—mainstream services, ethnically segregated services, and Eastern healing approaches.

Wong N: Psychiatric education and training of Asian and Asian-American psychiatrists. Am J Psychiatry 135:1525–1529, 1978

The Asian and Asian American physician training in a standard psychiatry residency is confronted both with discrimination at several levels and with special problems of professional role confusion and personal identity, creating barriers to professional development and productivity. The author proposes that general psychiatry residency programs establish a specialized track that focuses on ethnic minority groups. This approach may help improve the now inadequate resources for handling the mental health problems of Asian Americans and underuse of mental health resources by this group. Ethnic elderly patients are subsumed under the groups that might be helped by a broader pool of ethnic mental health professionals.

Conclusion

The stereotype of Asians as a well-adjusted model minority has been misleading with regard to the mental health of its elderly. The stereotype of the closely knit Asian family with reverence for elders, high economic assimilation, and low mental illness rates is untrue: there is a great deal of variation among Asian families. The current rise in the Asian population in the United States, including the elderly, reflects recent immigrants who are highly diverse in terms of customs, education, and resources. From the limited literature that exists on mental health in the Asian elderly, one can infer that culture shock, intergenerational strain, and lack of resources are intense problems for many Asian elderly individuals.

Interesting pilot work has shown possibilities of racial differences in psychiatric medication sensitivity and response, which must be followed up. Language barriers and limited financial resources, rather than cultural attitudes, often account for low service use. Data are inconclusive for higher rates of some disorders such as alcoholism or suicide, although these clinical perils are widely mentioned. Epidemiologic data on Asian elderly groups must be obtained, and further study of both heightened risk and protective factors for mental illness must be conducted, to plan culturally sensitive programs.

Appendix 1

References

Note. This reference list is organized, like the report, by ethnic minority group. It begins with a section of general references. The sections contain works cited in the text, works annotated in the chapter-section bibliographies, and additional works. The General References section and references with an asterisk (*) are not annotated in the text.

General References

Many articles and books on ethnic minority health and mental health do not focus on the elderly. We are including some of the more relevant general articles and books here that were not abstracted in the chapters. Some provide summaries of methodological issues or facts that have relevance to all age groups. Others are significant references that would not be discovered from computerized literature searches, either because they are chapters in books or because they are not indexed. Some old studies (over 15 years) are included because we feel they are still highly relevant.

American Association of Retired Persons: A Profile of Older Americans. Washington, DC, American Association of Retired Persons, 1985

Bengston VL, Cutler NE: Generations and intergenerational relations: perspectives on age groups and social change, in Handbook of Aging and the Social Sciences. Edited by Binstock R, Shanas E. New York, Van Nostrand Reinhold, 1976, pp 130–159

Chunn II JC, Dunston PJ, Ross-Sheriff F (eds): Mental Health and People of Color. Washington, DC, Howard University Press, 1983

Comas-Dias L, Griffith EEH (eds): Clinical Guidelines in Cross Cultural Mental Health. New York, Wiley, 1988

Dasen P, Sartonus N, Berry J (eds): Psychology, Culture, and Health: Toward Applications. Beverly Hills, CA, Sage, 1988

Flaskerund JH, Hu L: Racial/ethnic identity and amount and type of psychiatric treatment. Am J Psychiatry 149:379–384, 1992

Foulks EF, Wintrob RM, Westermeyer J, et al (eds): Current Perspectives in Cultural Psychiatry. New York, Spectrum Publications, 1977

Fry CL: Culture, behavior, and aging in the comparative perspective, in Handbook of the Psychology of Aging, 2nd Edition. Edited by Birren JE, Shaie KW. New York, Van Nostrand Reinhold, 1985, pp 216–244

Gaw A (ed): Cross-Cultural Psychiatry. Boston, MA, John Wright, 1982

Gaw AC: Culture, Ethnicity, and Mental Illness. Washington, DC, American Psychiatric Press, 1993

Giordano J: Ethnicity and Mental Health: Research and Recommendations. New York, Institute of Human Relations, 1973

Gorney R, Long M: Cultural determinants of achievement,aggression, and psychological distress. Arch Gen Psychiatry 37:452–459, 1980

Harper MS (ed): Minority Aging: Essential Curricula Content for Selected Health and Allied Health Professions (DHHS Publ No HRS-P-DV-90-4). Washington, DC, U.S. Government Printing Office, 1990

Health Resources and Services Administration: Health Status of Minorities and Low Income Groups (DHHS Publ No HRSA-HRS-P-DV 85-1). Rockville, MD, Health Resources and Services Administration, 1985

Ho MK: Family Therapy With Ethnic Minorities. Newbury Park, CA, Sage, 1987

Kendell RE, Cooper JE, Gourlay AJ, et al: The diagnostic criteria of American and British psychiatrists. Arch Gen Psychiatry 25:123–130, 1971

Kleinman A: Rethinking Psychiatry: From Cultural Category to Personal Experience. New York, Free Press, 1988

Lefley HP, Pedersen PB (eds): Cross-Cultural Training for Mental Health Professionals. Springfield, IL, Charles C Thomas, 1986

Malzberg B: Are immigrants psychologically disturbed? in Changing Perspectives in Mental Illness. Edited by Plog S, Edgerton R. New York, Holt, Rinehart & Winston, 1969, pp 395–421

Markides KS, Mindel CH: Aging and Ethnicity. Newbury Park, CA, Sage Publications, 1987

Markides KS, Liang J, Jackson JS: Race, ethnicity, and aging: conceptual and methodological issues, in Handbook of Aging and the Social Sciences, 3rd Edition. Edited by Binstock RH, George LK. New York, Academic, 1990, pp 112–129

Marsella AJ, Pederson PB (eds): Cross-Cultural Counseling and Psycho-therapy. New York, Pergamon, 1981

Marsella AJ, Sartorius N, Jablensky A, et al: Cross-cultural studies of depressive disorders: an overview, in Measurement of Depressive Disorders. Edited by Kleinman A, Good B. Berkeley, CA, University of California Press, 1985, pp 299–324

McGoldrick M, Pearce PK, Giordano J (eds): Ethnicity and Family Therapy. New York, Guilford, 1982

Moffic HS, Kendrick EA, Lomax JW, et al: Education in cultural psychiatry in the United States: overview. Transcultural Psychiatry Research 24:167–187, 1987

Office of the Assistant Secretary for Health: Healthy People 2000: National Health Promotion and Disease Prevention Objectives. Boston, MA, Jones and Bartlett Publishers, 1992

Price J: Foreign language interpreting in psychiatric practice. Austr N Z J Psychiatry 9:263–267, 1975

Rack P: Race, Culture, and Mental Disorder. New York, Tavistock, 1982

Rogler LH: The meaning of culturally sensitive research in mental health. Am J Psychiatry 146:296–303, 1989

Secretary's Task Force on Black and Minority Health: Report of the Secretary's Task Force on Black and Minority Health, Vol 1: Executive Summary (DHHS Publ No 491-313/44706). Washington, DC, Department of Health and Human Services, 1985

Sue DW, Due D: Counseling the Culturally Different: Theory and Practice, 2nd Edition. Somerset, NJ, Wiley, 1990

Triandis HC, Draguns JG (eds): Handbook of Cross-Cultural Psychology: Psychopathology, Vol 6. Boston, MA, Allyn & Bacon, 1980

United States Bureau of the Census: 1990 Census of Population: General Population Characteristics: U.S. Summary. Washington, DC, Department of Commerce, U.S. Bureau of the Census, U.S. Government Printing Office, 1990

United States Bureau of the Census: 1990 Census of Population and Housing Summary, Tape File 1C. Washington, DC, U.S. Department of Commerce, 1991

Wilkinson CB (ed): Ethnic Psychiatry. New York, Plenum Medical Book, 1986

World Health Organization: Dose effects of antidepressant medication in different populations: a WHO collaborative study. J Affect Dis (suppl 2, entire issue), 1986

Yager J, Chang C, Karno M: Teaching transcultural psychiatry. Academic Psychiatry 13:164–171, 1989

The African American Elderly

Adebimpe VR: Hallucinations and delusions in black psychiatric patients. J Natl Med Assoc 73:517–520, 1981

Adebimpe VR: Overview: white norms and psychiatric diagnosis of black patients. Am J Psychiatry 138:279–285, 1981

Baker FM: The black elderly: biopsychosocial perspective within an age cohort and adult development context. J Geriatr Psychiatry 15:227–239, 1982

Baker FM: The Afro-American life cycle: success, failure, and mental health. J Natl Med Assoc 79:625–633, 1987

Baker FM: Afro-Americans, in Clinical Guidelines in Cross Cultural Mental Health. Edited by Comas-Dias L, Griffith EEH. New York, Wiley, 1988, pp 151–181

Baker FM: Black youth suicide: literature review with a focus on prevention, in Report of the Secretary's Task Force on Youth Suicide, Vol 3: Prevention and Intervention in Youth Suicide (DHHS Publ No ADM-89-1623). Edited by Feinleib MR. Washington, DC, Alcohol, Drug Abuse, and Mental Health Administration, 1989, pp 177–195

Baker FM: Ethnic minority elders: differential diagnosis, medication, treatment, and outcomes, in Minority Aging: Essential Curricula Content for Selected Health and Allied Health Professions (DHHS Publ No HRS-P-DV-90-4). Edited by Harper MS. Washington, DC, U.S. Government Printing Office, 1990, pp 549–577

Baker FM: Dementing illness in African American populations: evaluation and management for the primary physicians. J Geriatr Psychiatry 24(1):73–91, 1991

Baker FM, Lightfoot OB: Psychiatric care of ethnic elders, in Culture, Ethnicity, and Mental Illness. Edited by Gaw AC. Washington, DC, American Psychiatric Press, 1993, pp 517–552

Baker FM, Lavizzo-Mourey R, Jones BE: Acute care of the African American elder. J Geriatr Psychiatry Neurol (in press)

Baker FM, Williams L, Bailey SF, et al: Black middle-class women in San Antonio, TX: coping strategies. J Natl Med Assoc 84(6):497–502, 1992

Baquet CR: Cancer prevention and control in the black population: epidemiology and aging implications, in The Black American Elderly: Research on Physical and Psychosocial Health. Edited by Jackson JS. New York, Springer, 1988, pp 50–68

Bell C, Mehte H: The misdiagnosis of black patients with manic-depressive illness. J Natl Med Assoc 72:141–145, 1979

Bell CC, Thompson JP, Lewis D, et al: Misdiagnosis of alcohol related organic brain syndromes: implications for treatment, in Treatment of Black Alcoholics. Edited by Brisbane FL, Womble M. New York, Haworth, 1985, pp 45–65

Bevis WM: Psychological traits of the Southern Negro with observations as to some of his psychoses. Am J Psychiatry 1:76–78, 1921

Bradshaw MH: Training psychiatrists for working with blacks in basic residency training programs. Am J Psychiatry 135:1520–1524, 1978

Brantley T: Racism and its impact on psychotherapy. Am J Psychiatry 140:1605–1608, 1983

Cannon M, Locke BZ: Being black is detrimental to one's mental health: myth or reality? Phylon 38:408–428, 1967

Carter JH: "Differential" treatment of the elderly black: victims of stereotyping. Postgrad Med 52:211–214, 1972

Carter JH: The black aged: implications for mental health care. J Am Geriatr Soc 30:67–70, 1982

Chatters LM, Taylor RJ, Jackson JS: Size and composition of the informal helper networks of elderly blacks. J Gerontol 40:605–614, 1985

Coner-Edwards AF, Spurlock J: Black Families in Crisis: The Middle Class. New York, Brunner/Mazel, 1988

Crawford FR: Variations between Negroes and whites in concepts of mental illness, its treatment, and prevalence, in Changing Perspectives in Mental Illness. Edited by Plog SS, Edgerton RB. New York, Holt, Rinehart & Winston, 1969, pp 242–256

Dana RH, Whatley PR: When does a difference make a difference? MMPI scores and African Americans. J Clin Psychol 47:400–406, 1991

Dancy Jr J: The Black Elderly: A Guide for Practitioners with Comprehensive Bibliography. Ann Arbor, MI, The Institute of Gerontology at the University of Michigan—Wayne State University, 1977

Drury TR, Powell AL: Prevalence of diabetes among black Americans, in Advance Data from Vital and Health Statistics, No 130 (DHHS Publ No PHS-87-1250). Hyattsville, MD, National Center for Health Statistics. Public Health Service, 1989

Gibson RC: Blacks in an Aging Society. New York, Carnegie Corporation, 1986

Griffith EEH, Young JL, Smith DL: An analysis of the therapeutic elements in a black church service. Hosp Community Psychiatry 35:464–469, 1984

Griffith EEH, Bell CC: Recent trends in suicide and homicide among blacks. JAMA 262:2265–2269, 1989

Gutman H: The Black Family in Slavery and Freedom. New York, Pantheon, 1976

Heisel MA, Faulkner A: Religiosity in an older black population. Gerontologist 22:354–358, 1982

Helzer J: Bipolar affective disorders in black and white men. Arch Gen Psychiatry 32:1140–1143, 1975

Hines PM, Boyd-Franklin N: Black families, in Ethnicity and Family Therapy. Edited by McGoldrick M, Pearce JK, Giordano J. New York, Guilford, 1982, pp 84–107

Jackson JJ: The blacklands of gerontology. Aging and Human Development 2:156–171, 1971

Jackson JJ: Sex and social class variations in black aged parent-child relationships. Aging and Human Development 2:96–107, 1971

Jackson JJ: "Help me somebody! I's an old black standing in the need of institutionalizing." Psychiatric Opinion 10:6–16, 1973

Jackson JJ: The plight of older black women in the United States. Black Scholar 7:47–55, 1976

Jackson JS: Growing old in black America: research on aging black populations, in The Black American Elderly: Research on Physical and Psychosocial Health. Edited by Jackson JJ. New York, Springer, 1988, pp 3–16

Jackson JS: Survey research in aging black populations, in The Black American Elderly: Research on Physical and Psychological Health. Edited by Jackson JS. New York, Springer, 1988, pp 327–346

Jackson JS (ed): Life in Black America. Newbury Park, CA, Sage, 1991

Jackson JS, Chatters L, Neighbors HW: The mental health status of older black Americans: a national study. Black Scholar 13:21–35, 1982

Jones A, Seagull A: Dimensions of the relationship between the black client and the white therapist. Am Psychol 32:850–855, 1977

Jones BE, Gray BA, Parson EB: Manic-depressive illness among poor urban blacks. Am J Psychiatry 1185:654–657, 1981

Jones BE, Gray BA, Jospitre J: Survey of psychotherapy with black men. Am J Psychiatry 139:1174–1177, 1982

Kramer M, Rosen M, Willis EM: Definition and distribution of mental disorders in a racist society, in Racism and Mental Health. Edited by Willie CV, Kramer BM, Brown BS. Pittsburgh, PA, University of Pittsburgh Press, 1973, pp 353–459

Lawson WB: Chronic mental illness and the black family. American Journal of Social Psychiatry 6:57–61, 1986

Lawson WB, Yesavage JA, Werner PA: Race, violence, and psychopathology. J Clin Psychiatry 45:294–297, 1984

Lewis JM, Looney JG: The Long Struggle: Well-Functioning Working Class Black Families. New York, Brunner/Mazel, 1983

Liss JL, Weiner A, Robins E, et al: Psychiatric symptoms in white and black inpatients. Compr Psychiatry 14:475–481, 1973

Manuel RC: The demography of older blacks in the United States, in The Black Elderly: Research on Physical and Psychosocial Health. Edited by Jackson JS. New York, Springer, 1988, pp 25–49

Martin EP, Marin JH: The Black Extended Family. Chicago, IL, University of Chicago Press, 1978

McAdoo H: Factors related to stability in upwardly mobile black families. Journal of Marriage and Family 40:761–776, 1978

Mullings L: Anthropological perspective of the Afro-American family, in The Black Family: Mental Health Perspectives. Edited by Fullilove MT. San Francisco, CA, Rosenberg Foundation, 1985, pp 11–21

Neighbors HW, Jackson JJ: The use of informal and formal help: four patterns of illness behavior in the black community. Am J Community Psychol 12:629–644, 1984

Pinderhughes CA: Racism and psychotherapy, in Racism and Mental Health. Edited by Willie CV, Kramer BM, Brown BS. Pittsburgh, PA, University of Pittsburgh Press, 1973, pp 61–121

Pinderhughes E: Afro-American families and the victim system, in Ethnicity and Family Therapy. Edited by McGoldrick M, Pearce JK, Giordano J. New York, Guilford, 1982, pp 108–122

Powell GJ: Overview of the epidemiology of mental illness among Afro-Americans, in The Afro-American Family: Assessment, Treatment, and Research Issues. Edited by Bass BA, Wyatt GE, Powell GJ. New York, Grune & Stratton, 1982, pp 155–163

President's Commission on Mental Health: Reports of Special Populations Subpanel on Mental Health of Black Americans, Vol 2 Appendix. Washington, DC, U.S. Government Printing Office, 1978

Raskin A, Crook TH, Herman KD: Psychiatric history and symptom differences in black and white depressed inpatients. J Consult Clin Psychol 43:73–80, 1975

Richardson J: Aging and Health: Black American Elders. Stanford, CA, Stanford Geriatric Education Center, 1990

Ruiz DS (ed): Handbook of Mental Health and Mental Disorders Among Black Americans. New York, Greenwood Press, 1990

Schachter J, Butts H: Transference and counter-transference in interracial analysis. J Am Psychoanal Assoc 16:792–909, 1968

Schoenberg BS, Anderson DW, Harer AF: Severe dementia: prevalence and clinical features in a biracial U.S. population. Arch Neurol 42:740–743, 1985

Seiden RH: Mellowing with age: factors influencing the non-white suicide rate. Int J Aging Hum Dev 13:265–284, 1981

Shader RI: Cultural aspects of mental health care for black Americans: cultural aspects of psychiatric training, in Cross-Cultural Psychiatry. Edited by Gaw A. Boston, MA, John Wright, 1982, pp 187–197

Simon RJ, Fleiss JL, Gurland BJ, et al: Depression and schizophrenic hospitalized black and white mental patients. Arch Gen Psychiatry 28:509–512, 1973

Sletten J, Schuff S, Altman H, et al: A statewide computerized psychiatric system: demographic, diagnostic, and mental status data. Int J Soc Psychiatry 18:30–40, 1972

Spurlock J: Black Americans, in Cross-Cultural Psychiatry. Edited by Gaw A. Boston, MA, John Wright, 1982, pp 163–178

Stack C: All Our Kin. New York, Harper & Row, 1974

Strickland TL, Ranganath V, Lin KM, et al: Psychopharmacologic considerations in the treatment of black American populations. Psychopharmacol Bull 27:441–448, 1991

Task Force on Black and Minority Health: Report on Black and Minority Health, Vol I: Executive Summary. Washington, DC, Department of Health and Human Services, 1985

Task Force on Black and Minority Health: Report on Black and Minority Health, Vol II: Cross-Cutting Issues in Minority Health. Washington, DC, Department of Health and Human Services, 1985

Task Force on Black and Minority Health: Report on Black and Minority Health, Vol III: Cancer. Washington, DC, Department of Health and Human Services, 1985

Task Force on Black and Minority Health: Report on Black and Minority Health, Vol IV: Cardiovascular and Cerebrovascular Disease, Part 2. Washington, DC, Department of Health and Human Services, 1985

Task Force on Black and Minority Health: Report on Black and Minority Health, Vol V: Homicide, Suicide, and Unintentional Injuries. Washington, DC, Department of Health and Human Services, 1985

Task Force on Black and Minority Health: Report on Black and Minority Health, Vol VI: Infant Mortality and Low Birthweight. Washington, DC, Department of Health and Human Services, 1985

Task Force on Black and Minority Health: Report on Black and Minority Health, Vol VII: Chemical Dependency and Diabetes. Washington, DC, Department of Health and Human Services, 1985

Taylor RJ: The extended family as a source of support to elderly blacks. Gerontologist 25:488–495, 1985

Taylor R, Chatters LM: Patterns of informal support to elderly black adults: family, friends, and church members. Soc Work 31:432–438, 1986

United States Bureau of the Census: Demographic aspects of aging and older populations in the United States, in Current Population Reports: Special Studies. Washington, DC, U.S. Government Printing Office, 1980

United States Bureau of the Census: Statistical Abstract of the United States: 1992, 112th Edition. Washington, DC, U.S. Department of Commerce, 1992

Valle R: U.S. ethnic minority groups' access to long-term care, in International Long Term Care. Edited by Meyers T. New York, McGraw-Hill, 1988, pp 339–365

Vitols MM, Water HG, Keeler MH: Hallucinations and delusions in white and Negro schizophrenics. Am J Psychiatry 120:472–476, 1963

Wilcox P: Positive mental health in the black community: the black liberation movement, in Racism and Mental Health. Edited by Willie CV, Kramer BK, Brown BS. Pittsburgh, PA, University of Pittsburgh Press, 1973, pp 463–482

Wylie FM: Attitudes toward aging black Americans: some historical perspectives. Aging and Human Development 2:66–70, 1971

The Hispanic American Elderly

Batista E: Sex-typed age norms among older Hispanics. Gerontologist 27:59–65, 1987

Bernstein IH, Teng G, Grannemann BD, et al: Invariance in the MMPI's components structure. J Pers Assess 54:522–531, 1987

Bird H, Canino G, Stipec MR, et al: Use of the Mini-Mental State Examination in a probability sample of Hispanic population. J Nerv Ment Dis 175:731–737, 1987

Bozlee S: A cross-cultural MMPI comparison of alcoholics. Psychol Rep 50:639–646, 1982

Bravo M, Canino GJ, Rubio-Stipec M, et al: A cross-cultural adaptation of a psychiatric epidemiologic instrument: the Diagnostic Interview Schedule's adaptation in Puerto Rico. Culture, Medicine, and Psychiatry 15:1–18, 1991

Burnam M, Hough R, Escobar J, et al: Six-month prevalence of specific psychiatric disorders among Mexican Americans and non-Hispanic whites in Los Angeles. Arch Gen Psychiatry 44:687–694, 1987

Burnam M, Hough R, Karno M, et al: Acculturation and lifetime prevalence of psychiatric disorders among Mexican Americans in Los Angeles. J Health Soc Behav 28:89–102, 1987

Castano R: Patterns and problems of drinking among U.S. Hispanics, in Report of the Secretary's Task Force on Black and Minority Health, Chemical Dependency and Diabetes, Vol VII. Washington, DC, Department of Health and Human Services, 1986

Comas-Dias L: Puerto Rican alcoholic women: treatment considerations. Alcoholism Treatment Quarterly 3:47–57, 1986

*Cuellar J: Aging and Health: Hispanic American Elders. Stanford, CA, Stanford Geriatric Education Center, 1990

Dolgin D, Grossner R, Cruz-Martinez S, et al: Discriminant analysis of behavioral symptomatology in hospitalized Hispanic and Anglo patients. Hispanic Journal of Behavioral Sciences 4:329–337, 1982

Escobar JI: Are results on the dexamethasone suppression test affected by ethnic background? Am J Psychiatry 142:268, 1985

Escobar JI, Burnham A, Karno M, et al: Use of the Mini-Mental State Examination in a community population of mixed ethnicity: cultural and linguistic artifacts. J Nerv Ment Dis 174:607–614, 1986

Espino DV, Neufeld RR, Mulvihill M, et al: Hispanic and non-Hispanic elderly on admission to the nursing home: a pilot study. Gerontologist 28:821–824, 1988

Franklin GS: Group psychotherapy for elderly female Hispanic outpatients. Hosp Community Psychiatry 33:385–387, 1982

Fuller CG, Malony HH: A comparison of English and Spanish (Nunez) translations of the MMPI. J Pers Assess 48:130–131, 1984

Furukawa C, Harris MB: Some correlates of obesity in the elderly: hereditary and environmental factors. Journal of Obesity and Weight Regulation 5:55–76, 1986

Garcia JL: A needs assessment of elderly Hispanics in an inner city senior citizen complex: implications for practice. J Appl Gerontol 4:72–85, 1985

Gaviria M, Stern G: Problems in designing and implementing culturally relevant mental health services for Latinos in the U.S. Soc Sci Med 14:65–71, 1980

Gonzalez DVA, Usher M: Group therapy with aged Latino women: a pilot project and study. Clinical Gerontologist 1:51–58, 1982

Greene MG, Adelman R, Charon R, et al: Ageism in the medical encounter: an exploratory study of the doctor-elderly patient relationship. Language Communication 6(1–2):113–124, 1986

Greene VL, Monahan DJ: Comparative utilization of community-based long-term care services by Hispanic and Anglo elderly in a case management system. J Gerontol 39:730–735, 1984

Guarnaccia P, Good B, Kleinman A: A critical review of epidemiological studies of Puerto Rican mental health. Am J Psychiatry 147:1449–1456, 1990

Hates-Bautista DE: Identifying "Hispanic" populations: the influence of research methodology upon public policy. Am J Public Health 70:353–356, 1980

Hoppe SK, Leon RL, Realini JP: Depression and anxiety among Mexican Americans in a family health center. Soc Psychiatry Psychiatr Epidemiol 24:63–68, 1989

Karno M: Acculturation and the probability of use of health services by Mexican Americans. Health Serv Res 24:238–257, 1989

Karno M, Hough R, Burnam M, et al: Lifetime prevalence of specific psychiatric disorders among Mexican Americans and non-Hispanic whites in Los Angeles. Arch Gen Psychiatry 44:695–701, 1987

Kemp BJ, Staples F, Lopez-Aqueres W: Epidemiology of depression and dysphoria in an elderly Hispanic population: prevalence and correlates. J Am Geriatr Soc 35:920–926, 1987

Kosten T, Rounsaville B, Kleber H: Ethnic and gender differences among opiate addicts. Int J Addict 20:1143–1162, 1985

Kutza EA: A policy analyst's response. Gerontologist 26:147–149, 1986

Lawrence RH, Bennett JM, Markides KS: Perceived intergenerational solidarity and psychological distress among older Mexican Americans. J Gerontol 47(social sciences suppl):S55–S65, 1992

Liang J, Tran VT, Krause N, et al: Generational differences in the structure of the CES-D in Mexican Americans. J Gerontol 44(social sciences suppl):S110–S120, 1989

Lopez-Aqueres W, Kemp B, Plopper M, et al: Health needs of the Hispanic elderly. J Am Geriatr Soc 32:191–198, 1984

Mahard RE: The CES-D as a measure of depressive mood in the elderly Puerto Rican population. J Gerontol 43:24–25, 1988

Maldonado D: The Hispanic elderly: a socio-historical framework for public policy. J Appl Gerontol 4:18–27, 1985

Malgady R, Rogler L, Constanino G: Ethnocultural and linguistic bias in mental health evaluation of Hispanics. Am Psychol 42:228–234, 1987

Marcos LR: Effects of interpreters on the evaluation of psychopathology in non-English speaking patients. Am J Psychiatry 136:171–174, 1979

Marcos L, Alpert M: Strategies and risks in psychotherapy with bilingual patients: the phenomenon of language independence. Am J Psychiatry 133:1275–1278, 1976

Marin BV, Marin G, Padilla AM, et al: Utilization of traditional and non-traditional sources of health care among Hispanics. Hispanic Journal of Behavioral Sciences 5:65–80, 1983

Markides KS, Coreil J: The health of Hispanics in the Southwest U.S.: an epidemiological paradox. Public Health Rep 101:253–265, 1986

Martinez Jr C: Mexican Americans, in Clinical Guidelines in Cross-Cultural Mental Health. Edited by Comas-Dias L, Griffith EEH. New York, Wiley, 1988, pp 151–181

Mendes deLeon C, Markides KS: Depressive symptoms among Mexican Americans: a three-generational study. Am J Epidemiol 127:150–160, 1988

Mindel CH: Extended familism among urban Mexican Americans, Anglos, and blacks. Hispanic Journal of Behavioral Sciences 2:21–34, 1980

Minrath M: Breaking the race barrier: the white therapist in interracial psychotherapy. J Psychosoc Nurs Ment Health Serv 23:19–24, 1985

Montgomery G, Orozco S: Mexican-Americans' performance on the MMPI as a function of the level of acculturation. J Clin Psychol 41:203–212, 1985

National Center for Health Statistics: Advance Report of Final Mortality Statistics (DHHS Publ No PHS-85-1120). Washington, DC, National Center for Health Statistics Monthly Vital Statistics Report 34(6, suppl 2), 1985

National Center for Health Statistics: Current Estimates from the National Health Interview Survey, U.S., in Vital and Health Statistics, Series 10 150 (DHHS Publ No PHS-85-1578). Washington, DC, National Center for Health Statistics, Public Health Service, U.S. Government Printing Office, 1985

National Center for Health Statistics: Health United States, 1985 (DHHS Publ No PHS-86-1232). National Center for Health Statistics. Washington, DC, U.S. Government Printing Office, 1985

Neff JR: Alcohol consumption and psychological distress among U.S. Anglos, Hispanics, and blacks. Alcohol Alcohol 21:111–119, 1986

Padilla A, Ruiz R: Latino Mental Health: A Review of the Literature. Rockville, MD, National Institute of Mental Health, 1973

Perez-Stable EI: Issues in Latino health care: medical staff conference. West J Med 146:213–218, 1987

Plemons G: A comparison of MMPI scores of Anglo- and Mexican-American psychiatric patients. J Consult Clin Psychol 45:149–150, 1987

Price CS, Cuellar I: Effects of language and related variables on the expression of psychopathology in Mexican American psychiatric patients. Hispanic Journal of Behavioral Sciences 3:145–160, 1981

Randolph ET, Escobar JI, Paz DH, et al: Ethnicity and reporting of schizophrenic symptoms. J Nerv Ment Dis 173:332–340, 1985

Smith JC, Mercy JA, Rosenberg ML: Suicide and homicide among Hispanics to health care and cuts in services: a state-of-the-art overview. Public Health Reports 101:238–252, 1986

Sokolovsky J: Ethnicity, culture and aging: do differences really make a difference? J Appl Gerontol 4:6–17, 1985

Swanda R, Kahn M: Differential perception of life crisis events by sex, diagnosis, and ethnicity in rural mental health clients. Journal of Rural Community Psychology 7:63–68, 1986

Szapocznik J, Lasagna J, Perry P, et al: Outreach in the delivery of mental health services to Hispanic elders. Hispanic Journal of Behavioral Sciences 1:21–40,1979

Szapocznik J, Santiseban D, Herris O, et al: Treatment of depression among Cuban-American elders: some validational evidence for a life enhancement counseling approach. J Consult Clin Psychol 49:752–754, 1981

Torres-Gil F: An examination of factors affecting future cohorts of elderly Hispanics. Gerontologist 26:140–146, 1986

Trevino FM (ed): Hispanic Health and Nutrition Examination Survey, 1982–1984: findings on health status and health care needs. Am J Public Health 80:(entire volume), 1990

Trevino FM, Moss AJ: Health indicators for Hispanic, black and white Americans, in Vital and Health Statistics, Series 10 148 (DHHS Publ No PHS-84-1576). Washington, DC, U.S. Government Printing Office, 1984

Tylim I: Group psychotherapy with Hispanic patients: the psychodynamics of idealization. Int J Group Psychother 32:339–350, 1982

United States Bureau of the Census: Projections of the Hispanic Population: 1983–2080 Population Estimates and Projections (series P-25, No 995). Washington, DC, U.S. Government Printing Office, 1986

United States Bureau of the Census: Nosotros. Washington, DC, Department of Commerce, 1985

United States Bureau of the Census: Persons of Spanish origin in the U.S.: March 1985, in Current Population Reports (series P-20, No 403). Washington, DC, Department of Commerce, 1985

*United States Bureau of the Census: Projections of the Hispanic Population: 1983–2080 Population Estimates and Projections (series P-25, No 995). Washington, DC, U.S. Government Printing Office, 1986

Vandenbos GR, Stapp J, Kilburg RR: Health service providers in psychology: results of the 1978 APA Human Resources Survey. Am Psychol 36:1403–1426, 1981

Vasquez C, Javier RA: The problem with interpreters: communicating with Spanish-speaking patients. Hosp Community Psychiatry 42:163–165, 1991

Ventura SJ: Births of Hispanic parentage. National Center for Health Statistics Monthly Vital Statistics Report 34(4 suppl), 1985

Weeks JR, Cuellar JB: Isolation of older persons: the influence of immigration and length of residence. Res Aging 5:369–388, 1983

Wells K, Hough R: Which Mexican Americans underutilize health services? Am J Psychiatry 144:918–922, 1987

Wetle T, Schensul J, Torres M, et al: Alzheimer's disease symptom interpretation and help-seeking among Puerto Rican elderly. Geriatric Education Center Newsletter, The University of Connecticut Travelers Center on Aging, 4(2), 1990

The American Indian Elderly

American Indian Nurses Association: Alternatives for Planning and Continuum of Care for Elderly American Indians. Final Report to Fulfill a Contract With the Indian Health Service. Rockville, MD, Indian Health Service, Public Health Service, Department of Health, Education, and Welfare, 1978

American Indian Nurses Association: The Environment of Elderly Native Americans. Final Report of a Contract With the Indian Health Service. Rockville, MD, Indian Health Service, U.S. Public Health Service, Department of Health, Education, and Welfare, 1978

Association of American Indian Physicians: Report on Physical and Mental Health of Elderly Indians. Final Report of a Contract With the Indian Health Service. Rockville, MD, Indian Health Service, U.S. Public Health Service, Department of Health, Education, and Welfare, 1978

Baron AE, Manson SM, Ackerson LM, et al: Depressive symptomatology in older American Indians with chronic disease: some psychometric considerations, in Screening for Depression in Primary Care. Edited by Attkisson C, Zich J. New York, Routledge, Chapman & Hall, 1990, pp 217–231

*Cuellar J: Aging and Health: American Indian/Alaskan Native. Stanford, CA, Stanford Geriatric Education Center, 1990

Focus on Native Health. Can Nurse 74(9):8–9, 1978

French J, Schwartz DR: Terminal care at home in two cultures. Am J Nurs 73:502–505, 1973

Goldstine T, Gutman D: A TAT study of Navajo aging. Psychiatry 35:373–384, 1972

Indian Health Service: Chart Book Series. Rockville, MD, Program Statistics Branch, Indian Health Service, Department of Health and Human Services (published annually)

Jelik WG, Todd N: Witchdoctors succeed where doctors fail: psychotherapy among the Coast Salish Indians. Canadian Psychiatric Association Journal 19:351–356, 1974

John R: Service needs and support networks of elderly Native Americans: family, friends, and social service agencies, in Social Bonds in Later Life: Aging and Interdependence. Edited by Peterson WA, Quadagno J. Beverly Hills, CA, Sage, 1985, pp 229–247

Joos SK, Ewart S: A health survey of Klamath Indian elders 30 years after the loss of tribal status. Public Health Rep 103:166–173, 1988

Kunitz SJ: Disease Change and the Role of Medicine: The Navajo Experience. Berkeley, CA, University of California Press, 1983

Kunitz SJ, Levy JE: A prospective study of isolation and mortality in a cohort of elderly Navajo Indians. Journal of Cross-Cultural Gerontology 3:71–85, 1988

Lewis TH: A syndrome of depression and mutism in the Oglala Sioux. Am J Psychiatry 132:753–755, 1975

Manson SM: Long-term care in American Indian communities: issues for planning and research. Gerontologist 29:38–44, 1989

Manson SM: Physicians and American Indian healers: issues and constraints in collaborative health care. (unpublished manuscript)

Manson SM: Provider assumptions about long-term care in American Indian communities. (unpublished manuscript)

Manson SM, Callaway DG: Problematic Life Situations: Cross-Cultural Variation in Support Mobilization Among the Elderly. Final report on Grant Number 0090-AR-0037. Administration on Aging, 1984

Manson SM, Callaway DG: Health and aging among American Indians: issues and challenges for the biobehavioral sciences, in Behavioral Health Issues Among American Indian and Alaska Natives: American Indian and Alaska Native Mental Health Research Monograph No 1. Edited by Manson SM, Dinges NG. Denver, CO, National Center for American Indian and Alaska Native Mental Health Research, 1988, pp 160–200

Manson SM, Heegard W: Urban Indian health care: the Portland program and patient population. Med Anthropol (in press)

Manson SM, Pambrun AM: Social and psychological status of the American Indian elderly: past research, current advocacy, and future inquiry. White Cloud Journal 1:18–25, 1979

Manson SM, Shore JH: Psychiatric epidemiological research among American Indians and Alaska Natives: methodological issues. White Cloud Journal 2:48–56, 1981

Manson SM, Shore JH, Bloom JD: The depressive experience in American Indian communities: a challenge for psychiatric theory and diagnosis, in Culture and Depression. Edited by Kleinman A, Good B. Berkeley, University of California Press, 1985, pp 331–368

Manson SM, Moseley R, Brenneman D: Physical illness, depression, and older American Indians: a preventive intervention trial, in Special Populations: Preventive Intervention Concerns: A New Beginning. Edited by Owan T, Silverman M. Washington, DC, U.S. Government Printing Office (in press)

May PA: Mental health and alcohol abuse indicators in the Albuquerque area of the Indian Health Service: an exploratory chart review. American Indian and Alaska Native Mental Health Research 2:33–46, 1988

Mick C: A Profile of American Indian Nursing Homes. Tucson, AZ, Working paper and reprint series, Long-Term Care Gerontology Center, University of Arizona, 1983

Montgomery RJ, Borgatta EF, Kamo Y, et al: A profile of Alaska's seniors: income, children, and health. Res Aging 10:534–549, 1988

National Indian Council on Aging: The Indian Elder: a Forgotten American—Final Report of the First National Indian Conference on Aging. Washington, DC, National Tribal Chairman's Association, 1976

National Indian Council on Aging: The Continuum of Life: Health Concerns of the Indian Elderly—Final Report of the Second National Indian Conference on Aging. Washington, DC, National Indian Council on Aging, 1978

National Indian Council on Aging: May the Circle Be Unbroken: A New Decade—Final Report on the Third National Indian Conference on Aging. Washington, DC, National Indian Council on Aging, 1980

National Indian Council on Aging: American Indian Elderly: A National Profile. Washington, DC, National Indian Council on Aging, 1981

National Indian Council on Aging: Indian Elders: A Tribute—Final Report of the Fourth National Indian Conference on Aging. Washington, DC, National Indian Council on Aging, 1982

Obomsawin R: A statement on Indian health. Can Nurse 74:7, 1978

Porter D: Mental health treatment and prevention: focus on elders, in Colloquium on American Indian Families: Developmental Strategies and Community Health. Edited by Mitchell W, Red Horse J. Phoenix, AZ, Arizona State University School of Social Work, 1982, pp 12–27

Rhoades ER, Marchall M, Attneave CL, et al: Impact of mental disorders upon elderly American Indians as reflected in visits to ambulatory care facilities. J Am Geriatr Soc 28:33–39, 1980

Shah CP, Farkas CS: The health of Indians in Canadian cities: a challenge to the health care system. Can Med Assoc J 133:859–863, 1985

Shomaker DJ: Transfer of children and the importance of grandmothers among the Navajo Indians. Journal of Cross-Cultural Gerontology 4:1–18, 1989

Shore JH, Manson SM: Cross-cultural studies of depression among American Indians and Alaska Natives. White Cloud Journal 2:5–12, 1981

Shore JH, Manson SM, Bloom JD, et al: A pilot study of depression among American Indian patients with Research Diagnostic Criteria. American Indian and Alaska Native Mental Health Research 1:4–15, 1987

Strong C: Stress and caring for elderly relatives: interpretations in coping strategies in an American Indian and white sample. Gerontologist 24:251–256, 1984

Surgeon General of the United States: Health Services for American Indians, Surgeon General's Report to Congress (PHS Publ No 531). Washington, DC, Public Health Service, Department of Health, Education, and Welfare, 1957

Taylor TL: Health problems and use of services at two urban American Indian clinics. Public Health Rep 103:88–95, 1988

Timpson JB: Indian mental health: challenges in the delivery of care in northwestern Ontario. Can J Psychiatry 29:234–241, 1984

United States Congress, Office of Technology Assessment: Indian Health Care (Publ No OTA-H-290). Washington, DC, U.S. Government Printing Office, 1986

Westermeyer J, Walker D, Benton E: A review of some methods for investigating substance abuse among American Indians and Alaska Natives. White Cloud Journal 2:13–21, 1981

White House Conference on Aging: Report on the Special Concerns Session on the Elderly Indian. Washington, DC, U.S. Government Printing Office, 1971

White House Conference on Aging: The American Indian and Alaska Native Elderly. Technical Report. Washington, DC, U.S. Government Printing Office, 1981

Young TK: Self-perceived and clinically assessed health status of Indians in Northwestern Ontario: analysis of a health survey. Can J Public Health 73:272–277, 1982

The Asian and Pacific American Elderly

Babcock CG, Gehrie MJ: Psychoanalysis and follow-up: the personal and cultural meaning of the experience of Nisei in treatment (NIMH Fellowship Grant No 5-F22-MH02492-01,02 03). Paper presented at the Research Meeting of the Chicago Institute for Psychoanalysis, March 24, 1977

Biser M: Influences of time, ethnicity, and attachment on depression in Southeast Asian refugees. Am J Psychiatry 145:46–51, 1988

Braun KL, Humphrey JW, Kaku JM: Community long-term care for geriatric patients in Hawaii. Hawaii Med J 46:417–431, 1987

*Chan S: Asian Americans: An Interpretive History. Boston, MA, Twayne Publishers, 1983

Chen P: A study of Chinese-American elderly residing in hotel rooms. Soc Casework 60:89–95, 1979

Cox C: Physician utilization by three groups of ethnic elderly. Med Care 24:667–676, 1986

Fujii SM: Elderly Asian Americans and use of public services. Soc Casework 57:202–207, 1976

Gozdiak E: What providers need to know to serve older refugees. The Aging Connection (The American Society on Aging newsletter), April/May 1990, pp 7, 10

Group for the Advancement of Psychiatry (GAP), Committee on Cultural Psychiatry: Suicide and Ethnicity in the United States (Report No 128). New York, Brunner/Mazel, 1989

Hayes CL: Two worlds in conflict: the elderly Hmong in the United States, in Ethnic Dimensions of Aging. Edited by Gelfand DE, Barrest CM. New York, Springer, 1987, pp 79–95

Hing E: Use of nursing homes by the elderly: preliminary data from the 1985 nursing home survey (DHHS Publ No PHS-87-1250), Advance Data from Vital and Health Statistics No 135. Hyattsville, MD, Public Health Service, 1987

Hughes GW: Neuropsychiatric aspects of bilingualism: a brief review. Br J Psychiatry 139:25–28, 1981

Ibrahim IB, Carter C, McLaughlin D, et al: Ethnicity and suicide in Hawaii. Soc Biol 24:10–16, 1977

Kalish RA: Suicide: an ethnic comparison in Hawaii. Bulletin of Suicidology 4:37–43,1968

Kiefer CW, Kim S, Choi K, et al: Adjustment problems of Korean American elderly. Gerontologist 24:477–482, 1985

Kinzie DJ, Manson SM, Vuh DT, et al: Development and validation of a Vietnamese-language depression rating scale. Am J Psychiatry 139:1276–1281, 1982

Kitano HL: Japanese-American mental illness, in Changing Perspectives in Mental Illness. Edited by Plog SS, Edgerton RB. New York, Holt, Rinehart & Winston, 1969, pp 256–284

Kitano HL, Daniels R: Asian Americans: Emerging Minorities. Englewood Cliffs, NJ, Prentice-Hall, 1988

Koh S, Sakauye KM, Koh TH: Adaptive capabilities of newly immigrated Asian elderly. Quarterly Contact 4:3, 1981

Koh S, Sakauye KM, Koh TH, et al: A reflection on the study of Asian American elderly by Asian American researchers. Asian American Psychological Association Journal 8:22–23, 1983

Kuo W: Theories of migration and mental health: an empirical testing on Chinese-Americans. Soc Sci Med 10:297–306, 1976

Kuo WH: Prevalence of depression among Asian-Americans. J Nerv Ment Dis 172:449–457, 1984

Kuo WH: Social networking, hardiness, and immigrant's mental health. J Health Soc Behav 27:133–149, 1986

Lin KM: Hwa-Byung: a Korean culture-bound syndrome? Am J Psychiatry 140:105–107, 1983

Lin KM, Tazuma L, Masuda M: Adaptational problems of Vietnamese refugees; I: health and mental health status. Arch Gen Psychiatry 36:955–961, 1979

Lin KM, Poland RE, Smith MW, et al: Pharmacokinetic and other related factors affecting psychotropic responses in Asians. Psychopharmacol Bull 27:427–440, 1991

Lin TY, Lin MC: Service delivery issues in Asian-North American communities. Am J Psychiatry 135:454–456, 1978

Liu WT: Health services for Asian elderly. Res Aging 8:156–175, 1986

Liu WT, Yu E: Asian/Pacific American elderly: mortality differentials, health status, and use of health services. J Appl Gerontol 4:35–64, 1985

Liu WT, Lamanna M, Murata A: Transition to Nowhere: Vietnamese Refugees in America. Nashville, TN, Charter House, 1979

Lyman SM: Chinese Americans. New York, Random House, 1974

Marsella AJ, Kameoka VA: Ethnocultural issues in the assessment of psychopathology, in Measuring Mental Illness: Psychometric Assessment for Clinicians. Edited by Wetzler S. Washington, DC, American Psychiatric Press, 1989, pp 229–256

Masuda M, Lin KM, Tazuma L: Adaptational problems of Vietnamese Refugees; II: life changes and perception of life events. Arch Gen Psychiatry 37:447–450, 1980

Matsushima NM, Tashima N: Mental Health Treatment Modalities of Pacific/Asian American Practitioners (NIMH Grant No 1-RO1 MH32148), A Report of the Pacific Asian Mental Health Research Project, San Francisco, CA, 1982

McIntosh JL, Santos JF: Suicide among minority elderly: a preliminary investigation. Suicide Life Threat Behav 11:151–166, 1981

Moon A, Tashima N: Help-seeking Behavior and Attitudes of Southeast Asian Refugees (Funded by NIMH Grant No 1-RO1 MH32148). San Francisco, CA, Pacific Asian Mental Health Research Project, 1982

Morioka-Douglas N, Yeo G: Aging and Health: Asian/Pacific Island American Elders. Stanford, CA, Stanford Geriatric Education Center, 1990

Nahirny VC, Fishman JA: American immigrant groups: ethnic identification and the problem of generations. Sociol Rev 13:311–326, 1965

Nandi PK: The Quality of Life of Asian Americans: An Exploratory Study in a Middle-Size Community. Chicago, IL, Pacific-American Mental Health Resource Center, 1980

National Pacific/Asian Resource Center on Aging: Pacific/Asian Elderly Bibliography. Seattle, WA, National Pacific/Asian Resource Center on Aging, 1980

Office of Disease Prevention and Health Promotion: Disease Prevention/Health Promotion: The Facts—U.S. Public Health Service. Palo Alto, CA, Bull Publishing Co, 1986

Osako MM: Japanese Americans: melting into the all-American pot? in Ethnic Chicago. Edited by Jones d'A, Hilli MG. Grand Rapids, MI, Eerdmans, 1983, pp 314–344

Peterson MR, Rose CL, McGee RI: A cross-cultural health study of Japanese and Caucasian Asians in Hawaii. Int J Aging Hum Dev 21:267–279, 1985

Rahe RH, Looney JG, Ward HW, et al: Psychiatric consultation in a Vietnamese refugee camp. Am J Psychiatry 135:185–190, 1978

Sakauye KM: Ethnic variations in family support of the frail elderly, in Family Involvement in Treatment of the Frail Elderly. Edited by Zucker-Goldstein M. Washington, DC, American Psychiatric Press, 1989, pp 63–106

Sata LS: A profile of Asian-American psychiatrists. Am J Psychiatry 135:448–454, 1978

Sauna VD: Immigration and mental illness: a review of the literature with special emphasis on schizophrenia, in Behavior in New Environments. Edited by Brody E. Beverly Hills, CA, Sage, 1969, pp 291–352

*Srole L, Langner T, Michael S, et al: Mental Health in the Metropolis: The Midtown Manhattan Study. New York, McGraw-Hill, 1962

Stavig GR, Igra A, Leonard AR: Hypertension and related health issues among Asians and Pacific Islanders in California. Public Health Rep 103:28–37, 1988

Uba L: Meeting the mental health needs of Asian Americans: mainstream or segregated services. Professional Psychology 12:215–221, 1982

United States Census Bureau of the Census: Asian and Pacific Islander population in the United States: 1980, in 1980 Census of Population, Vol 2, Special Reports, 1988

United States Bureau of the Census: We the Asian and Pacific Islander Americans. Washington, DC, U.S. Bureau of the Census, 1988

Valle R: Natural support systems, minority groups, and the late life dementias: implications for service delivery, research, and policy, in Clinical Aspects of Alzheimer's Disease and Senile Dementia (Aging, Vol 15). Edited by Miller NE, Cohen GD. New York, Raven, 1981, pp 277–299

Weinstein-Shr G: Breaking the Linguistic and Social Isolation of Refugee Elders: An Intergenerational Model. (personal communication, 1988)

Westermeyer J: Psychiatric diagnosis across cultural boundaries. Am J Psychiatry 142:798–805, 1985

Wong N: Psychiatric education and training of Asian and Asian-American psychiatrists. Am J Psychiatry 135:1525–1529, 1978

Wu F: Mandarin-speaking aged Chinese in the Los Angeles area. Gerontologist 15:271–275, 1975

Yamamoto J, Wagatsuma H: The Japanese and Japanese Americans. Journal of Operational Psychiatry 11:120–1335, 1980

Yamamoto J, Machizawa S, Araki F, et al: Mental health of elderly Asian Americans in Los Angeles. American Journal of Social Psychiatry 5:37–46, 1985

Yamamoto J, Yamamoto M, Steinberg A, et al: Alcohol abuse among elderly Asians in Los Angeles: a pilot study. Pacific/Asian American Mental Health Research Center Research Review 6:26–27, 1988

Yu E, Liu WT, Kurzeja P: Physical and mental health status indicators for Asian/Pacific Americans—Subreport prepared for the Report of the Secretary's Task Force on Black and Minority Health. Washington, DC, U.S. Government Printing Office, 1985

Appendix 2

Resources

General Resources

Minority Affairs Initiative
Health and Ethnicity Committee
American Association of Retired
  Persons (AARP)
1909 K Street, NW
Washington, DC 20006
(202) 434-2277

Minority Concerns Committee
National Task Force on Minority
  Elders
National Low Income Elder
  Initiative
American Society on Aging
833 Market Street, Suite 512
San Francisco, CA 94103
(415) 882-2910

Technical Assistance Program Director
Task Force on Minority Issues
The Gerontological Society
1275 K Street, NW, Suite 305
Washington, DC 20005
(202) 842-1275

African American Elderly

Michelle O. Clark, M.D.
The Black Task Force
Department of Psychiatry
San Francisco General Hospital
San Francisco, CA 94110
(415) 206-8000

National Caucus and Center on
  Black Aged
1424 K Street, NW
Washington, DC 20005
(202) 637-8400

National Resource Center on
  Minority Aging Populations
University Center on Aging
College of Health and Human
  Services
San Diego State University
San Diego, CA 92182
(619) 594-6765

Susan A. Schoenrock, M.P.H.
Editor, *Minority Aging Exchange*
Newsletter of the National
  Resource Center on Minority
  Aging Populations (NRCMAP)
Center on Aging
College of Health and Human
  Services
San Diego State University
San Diego, CA 92182
(619) 594-5200

Hispanic American Elderly

Gerontological Researchers

Elias Anzola-Perez, M.D.
Regional Advisor
Health Care for the Elderly
Pan American Health Organization
World Health Organization
525 23rd Street
Washington, DC 20037
(202) 861-3273

Elene Bastida, Ph.D.
Associate Professor
Department of Sociology and
  Social Work
Wichita State University
Wichita, KS 67260
(316) 689-3456

Marjorie Cantor, Ph.D.
Director
Brookdale Institute on Aging
Fordham University
Lincoln Center
New York, NY 10023-7479
(212) 636-6000

Rumaldo Juarez, Ph.D.
Associate Professor
Department of Sociology and
  Social Work
Pan American University
Edinburg, TX 78539
(210) 381-2011

Rita Mahard
Hispanic Research Center
Fordham University
Bronx, NY 10454
(212) 636-6000

Kyriakos Markides, Ph.D.
Professor
School of Public Health
University of Texas Medical Branch
Houston, TX 77030
(713) 792-2121

Juan Orcesitas, M.D.
Center on Adult Development
  and Aging
1425 NW 10th Avenue
Sieron Building
Suite 200
Miami, FL 33136
(305) 326-1043

Maribel Taussig, Ph.D.
Andrus Gerontology Center
University Park ML 0191
University of Southern California
Los Angeles, CA 90089-0191
(213) 743-8123

Ramon Valle, Ph.D.
Hispanic Community Research
    Project
University of San Diego
6506 Alvarado, Suite 112
San Diego, CA 92182
(619) 286-7151

Policy Researchers in Gerontology

Manual Miranda, Ph.D.
330 Independence Avenue, SW
Suite 4760
Washington, DC 20201
(202) 619-0724

Fernando Torres-Gil, Ph.D.
Andrus Gerontology Center
University Park ML 0191
University of Southern California
Los Angeles, CA 90089-0191
(213) 740-2311

Asian and Pacific American Elderly

The National Asian Pacific
    Center on Aging
Don Watanabe, Executive Director
Melbourne Tower, Suite 914
1511 Third Avenue
Seattle, WA 98121
(206) 624-1221

Edmond Pi, M.D.
Director
U.S.C. Medical Center
Asian Inpatient Psychiatry Unit
1934 Hospital Place
Los Angeles, CA 90033
(213) 226-5623

Stanley Sue, Ph.D.
Asian Mental Health Research
    Center
University of California at Los
    Angeles
Department of Psychology
Los Angeles, CA 90024-1563
(310) 825-3140

Keh-Ming Lin, M.D.
Associate Professor of Psychiatry
Harbor-UCLA Medical Center
Department of Psychiatry
1000 West Carson Street
Torrance, CA 90509
(310) 533-2345

Index

*Page numbers printed in **boldface** type refer to tables.*

in access to mental health
services, 43
in families, 50
in manic-depressive disorder,
31–32
in mental health status, 34–35
Asian/Pacific Americans, 119,
124–125
Hispanic Americans, 80–81
family income, 65
in use of health care services, 84
Somatization, 16, 121
Southeast Asians
culture-bound syndromes, 121
depression in, 129
Southwest U.S., 74, 75, 78–79
Spanish
screening tests, 74, 75
transference and idealization and,
87–88
Standard errors in Epidemiologic
Catchment Area studies, 15
Stereotyping of African Americans,
44, 56–59, 62
Substance abuse. *See* Alcohol abuse;
Drug abuse
Suicide
in African Americans, 24
in American Indians, 98
in Asian/Pacific Americans, 122,
125–127
in Hispanic Americans, 79
of whites versus non-whites, 55
Support network
African Americans, 50–56, 59–60
American Indians, 109–111
Asian/Pacific Americans, 126,
132–134, 140
Hispanic Americans, 81–82
"Survivor effect," 3

T
Terminally ill in Navajo versus Italian
culture, 106–107
Thematic Apperception Test (TAT),
98
Therapy. *See* Treatment
Toxic chemicals and African
Americans, 56
Tranquilizers, 32
Transference, 58, 87–88
Treatment
African Americans
cultural values in, 44
family therapy, 54
interracial therapeutic
relationship, 56–59
medical, 37
psychotherapy, 37, 40–41, 54
American Indians, 112
Asian/Pacific Americans, **139,** 144
Hispanic Americans, 86–89
racial differences in, 3
racism and, 40, 43–44

U
U.S. population
African Americans, 22
all ages and elders, **5**
Asian/Pacific Americans, 116
elders, **7,** 26
Hispanic Americans, **6,** 64, **65**

V
"Victim system," 26
Vietnamese
adaptational problems, 141–142
depression in, 129–130
health and mental health status,
141–142
health service use, 137